M000115534

What People Are Saying in Prais[...]

"This tremendous resource will shift your paradigm about healthcare. It's simple, eye-opening, and fun to read! When conventional medicine hasn't entirely provided the answers you're looking for, it may be time to think outside of the box and consider the possibility that nature may have already long-since provided remedies for many of the ailments that plague society today. So sit back and enjoy these stories from real people who struggled with real challenges, and the fascinating ways in which they overcame them."

~Leslie Householder, bestselling author of The Jackrabbit Factor: Why You Can, www.jackrabbitfactor.com

"I've always been a huge believer in the power of personal stories in setting others on the path to wellness. The 25 "Natural Medicine Confessions" shared in **Trust Your Intuition** are all very different, yet very similar. These women have used what they have learned to heal themselves and their family members. The results of their "mama bear" instincts coming out are simply amazing and inspiring! While I'm already familiar with the benefits of dietary changes in healing and becoming our best possible selves, there was much more to learn from this book. I plan to reference these stories and the wisdom in them from this point on. Therefore, this book will be highlighted and notated, and "at the ready" at my home from this point on. Many thanks to all who so graciously shared their stories and what they have learned, so that the rest of us might benefit."

~Shirley Braden, author at www.glutenfreeeasily.com

"Confidence in your chosen path is critical if you're going to succeed in a natural health treatment that runs against what most of society follows. If you need a dose of confidence, Trust Your Intuition will give you just that—example after example of people who have used real food, natural medicine and trust in their body's design to overcome health challenges. As someone who was left for dead by the conventional medicine doctors, I understand how hard it is to find your own answers. I applaud these women for their bravery in taking control of their health or the health of their family members. Swimming upstream is incredibly difficult, and these women show you how you can do it successfully."

~KerryAnn, author at Cooking Traditional Foods, www.cookingtf.com

"From dealing with common childhood illnesses, to chronic adult diseases, to losing weight, to creating natural medicine cabinets, to treating our four-legged friends—Trust Your Intuition is a must-have book for fresh and seasoned natural health enthusiasts. It's less like a book and more like reading stories from some of the best natural health bloggers on the web, each of which inspire and instruct on a variety of topics sure to peak your interest when it comes to healthy living and encouraging you to truly trust your intuition."

Meagan Visser—Blog Editor: Bulk Herb Store

"It's easy to feel frustrated with America's 'health care' (i.e. 'sick care') system that mostly treats symptoms and ignores root causes. But in this excellent, well-researched, and thorough book, Jenni Wilson shows that we don't have to be frustrated—we can be empowered to bypass the flaws in the system and administer true health in our own homes. As the wife of a MD, Jenni bridges the divide between traditional and natural medicine with grace and ease. This is not a typical angry rant, but a credible and sincere source of legitimate solutions. Jenni and her contributors have proven themselves to be trustworthy thought leaders in health and wellness, and anyone who cares about the health of their family should read and apply the principles in this fabulous book."

~Stephen Palmer, Founder of LifeManifestos.com, Author of *Uncommon Sense: A Common Citizen's Guide to Rebuilding America*

Trust Your Intuition

Trust Your Intuition

25 "Natural Medicine Confessions"
From Influential Women Who Use
Healing Remedies For Their Families

JENNI WILSON, M.H.

Copyright © 2013 by JENNI WILSON, M.H.

ISBN: Softcover   978-1-4836-3755-6
          Ebook   978-1-4836-3756-3

All rights reserved. No part of this book may be reproduced or transmitted in any form or by any means, electronic or mechanical, including photocopying, recording, or by any information storage and retrieval system, without permission in writing from the copyright owner.

This book was printed in the United States of America.

Disclaimer
Nothing in this book claims to diagnose, cure, or prevent any disease. This book is a tool for helping people take more responsibility for their own health. This book is not a substitute for conventional medical care, but is an educational resource.

Trademarks
Any trademarks mentioned herein are the property of their respective owners.

Rev. date: 06/04/2013

To order additional copies of this book, contact:
Xlibris Corporation
1-888-795-4274
www.Xlibris.com
Orders@Xlibris.com
113488

Contents

Foreword..13
—By Michael L. Wilson, M.D

A Note From Jenni...17

How Did An MD Husband and Master Herbalist Wife
    Come To Terms About Medicine? 19
—By Jenni Wilson, http://www.MomEssentials.net, http://www.NaturalMedicineMom.com

Back to Basics: Using Natural Tools to Heal Colds and Ear Infection....26
—By Katie, http://www.wellnessmama.com

Conventional Medicine Left Me Helpless.............................33
—By Patty Lacoss-Arnold, http://www.lovingourguts.com

It's True! We Lost Fat by Eating MORE Fat!........................40
—By Kate Tietje, http://www.ModernAlternativeMama.com

Addressing ADHD with Alternatives..................................46
—By Penny Williams, http://www.adhdmomma.com

How We Went From Morbidly Obese to Making Changes
    That Saved My Husband's Life.................................52
—By Brandie Schwartz, CHHC, AADP, RNWCON, http://www.eatyourselftolife.com

From Infertile to A Beautiful Baby Girl: How I Conceived
    Naturally When My Doctors Told Me I Couldn't..........59
—By Mare Pulido, http://www.holisticmamas.com

Red Raspberry Tea: A Woman's Best Friend 66
—By Paula J. Miller, http://www.wholeintentions.com

Proud, Strong, and Confident: Why I Decided To Go
  With a Natural Birth 74
—*By Cara Nitz, http://www.yourworldnatural.blogspot.com*

Mama Goes Natural: Plus Bonus Tips & Recipes 81
—*By Kristy Howard, http://www.littlenaturalcottage.com*

From Intimidated to Empowered 91
—*By Jill Winger, http://www.theprairiehomestead.com*

Recipes for Success: Cough Syrup, Lung Formula,
  Congestion, and Respiratory Sicknesses.........................98
—*By Jill of Jill's Home Remedies, http://www.jillshomeremedies.com*

Fighting a Fever? Think Again....................................108
—*By Sara Shay, http://www.YourThrivingFamily.com*

Did Someone Just Say 'LICE?' My Tips To Getting Rid of Nits Naturally 116
—*By Kelly Moeggenborg, http://www.kellythekitchenkop.com*

Addressing Crohn's Disease by Cutting Carbs? 124
—*By Vicky, http://www.glutenfreescdandveggie.blogspot.co.uk*

Healthy Gut, Healthy Child.......................................130
—*By Stacy S. Hirsch, http://www.totheroot.com, http://www.stacyhirsch.com*

How I Healed My Son's Skin Infection Without Antibiotics 138
—*By Stephanie Langford, http://www.keeperofthehome.org*

No More Vics, Vapo, Vaccines, and Vegetarianism—
  How I Trusted My Intuition......................................144
—*By Stacy Karen, http://www.adelightfulhome.com*

Fat to Fast—How I Changed My Life to Get Off my Couch
  and Into a 5K in Only 6 Weeks! 152
—*By Gina Mooney, http://www.slowisthenewfast.com*

A Mother's Journey to Natural Living.............................158
—*By Sara Elizabeth, http://www.amamasstory.com*

Secret Go-To Infection Formula From A Successful,
    Fashion-Designing Mom...166
    —*By Corinne Rickenbach, http://www.PersnicketyClothing.com*

My Change of Heart that took me from Medical School
    to a World Expert in Natural Medicine 172
    —*By Pina LoGiudice ND, LAC, http://www.innersourcehealth.com*

Saving Bruno: How I Used Natural Remedies to Heal My 4-Legged Baby.... 178
    —*By Laurie Driggers, http://www.inspiredhealthandhappiness.com*

Taking Health Into My Own Hands: How Acne Brought Me Gratitude 185
    —*By Robin Konie, http://www.thankyourbody.com*

Maximize your Living!...191
    —*By Rachel Marie, http://www.day2dayjoys.com*

Epilogue 199

Acknowledgements

I am immensely grateful for wonderful women authors who are contributing to this book. Each one is a leader and educator, passionate about educating the masses, teaching principles of health and happiness in her own personal way. I respect them all enormously and am impressed by their stories of determination, persistence and grit. I am so happy that they agreed to take part in this book! I know my readers will be too, as this collection is truly fantastic! I want to give my thanks to each contributor for her efforts and patience, as the editing of the project took longer than expected.

I don't know how I could have even thought about doing this project without the love, help and support of my sweet husband, Mike. He has my gratitude for his great patience through all of my endeavors and for keeping our home from turning into an absolute circus through my busiest times. I love him dearly. He has truly given me wings to fly.

To my wonderful children, Nathaniel, Raquel, Isaac, Seth, Liliana, Joel and Ian, who have inspired me to seek for healthy solutions in our family, allowed me to practice on them a wide variety of remedies, and who have endured with patience my many hours at the computer.

I want to thank my assistants, Lisa Childs and Brooke Bomar, for their invaluable help and especially Lisa for her organization skills, professional opinion and ability to keep track of all the tiny details. Thanks goes to Nancy Chrisovergi for her gorgeous cover design and for being so easy to work with. I'm grateful to my sister, Emili (emiliwhitneyphotography. com), for capturing the beautiful photo of my baby and I for the front cover.

To my friends, family and readers who continue to give me so much love and encouragement. It fires my passion onward for empowering families in whole medicine and good health.

Foreword

By Michael L. Wilson, M.D.

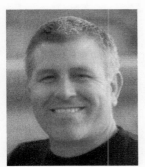

I'm an Emergency Medicine Physician. It is 3:00 am. Tonight in the ER there is a drunk male in the police holding room, a middle aged woman with chest pain in the cardiac room, and a three-year old with a fever waiting to be seen. His mother brings him in because he woke up coughing and "felt hot," so she wanted to make sure he is okay.

He played all day with his cousins and went to bed happy and comfortable. I walk in the room and he is smiling and laughing and has a temperature of 101.5 degrees. His mother indicates he seems to be feeling better, has not thrown up, and when asked if she has given him anything for the fever, she says "no, I just was worried and scared, so I brought him here".

Fear and lack of knowledge underlie why most people seek emergency medical care. This fear is a result of not taking time or making the effort to learn more about their own health, or the health of their family. Ignorance drives fear and saps us of power to make effective and wise choices. As we remember from Schoolhouse Rock, "Knowledge is Power." Ignorance creates a dependence on others and results in powerlessness.

The "natural," "alternative," "integrative," "complementary," or "holistic" health revolution that is occurring can cause scoffing and at times derision among conventional health providers and systems, but it also results in a more informed, responsible, and healthier group of individuals and families.

Women are at the forefront of this movement. They often are more willing (at times forced) to take responsibility for the health and welfare of themselves and their families. They often are more connected with their children's health needs, diet, and discomforts. Often, alternative natural therapies and philosophies appeal to women because they have experienced their own health challenges and have sought answers through conventional channels, only to be told that nothing is wrong.

As a conventional medical practitioner, I see the deterioration of our current model of health care (a misnomer: it is actually "sick care") and I see that this model is unsustainable.

There are multiple areas of technological innovation that have been designed to increase the quality of health care, but often result merely in the ability to diagnose the problem, without having a good solution besides treating the symptoms.

Modern conventional medicine is great at two things:

1. Surgical emergencies, including traumatic injuries
2. Acute disease processes like heart attacks and breathing failure

Chronic problems are a challenge because many of these are caused over decades of treating one's body poorly, intentionally or unknowingly. These problems cannot be "fixed" with simple chemical medical treatments; they require lifestyle changes that require the thing conventional medicine isn't good at: empowerment, knowledge, true innovation and questioning current ways of providing care.

The true innovators in health care are those who currently are on the outside looking in, being pushed and promoted often by women who are dissatisfied by the medical status quo and who *want* to **take** responsibility for their health and that of their families.

Women are also the true providers of *health care*. By promoting healthy diets and exercise for themselves and their families, by educating themselves about natural and alternative remedies that are less toxic and often more effective for non-life-threatening problems (like non-specific abdominal pain, fevers with cold symptoms, non-specific cough, nausea, vomiting, and migraines), women are taking control of health care at home.

H. Gilbert Welch, at Dartmouth Medical School describes it this way:

"For years now, people have been encouraged to look to medical care as the way to make them healthy. But that's your job—you can't contract that out. Doctors might be able to help, but so might an author of a good cookbook, a personal trainer, a cleric or a good friend. We would all be better off if the medical system got a little closer to its original mission of helping sick patients, and let the healthy be." (1)

Even in interactions with the medical system, intuition plays an important role. A friend in Uruguay was concerned about her daughter's lack of energy and generalized complaints. With research and her own "feelings" Alexandra took her child to the physician, telling her she thought her daughter had diabetes. Condescendingly came the response: "And what makes you think she has diabetes?"

Three hours later, the young girl was diagnosed with diabetes. Fast forward one year, almost to the date: Alexandra again felt that something just wasn't right with her daughter. She took the day off work to stay home with her. Her daughter had her first diabetic seizure that day. This mother was so grateful to have that intuition and to have paid attention to that inner voice.

This intuitive, loving woman also has a son with autism and is looking for alternative interventions for her son because of the disagreements and infighting among the physicians who have seen her child. She really wants more information so that she can trust herself to know what her son needs.

There are many other women out there just like her.

So bring on the intuition. Bring on the innovation and cost savings. Bring on the healthier families, individuals, and communities that result from women taking back responsibility for their own health care and the health care of their families. Go ahead ladies. Trust your intuition.

It is easy to get a thousand prescriptions but hard to get one single remedy.

~Chinese Proverb

A Note From Jenni

I had a health crisis while my husband, Mike, was in medical school. I had been seeing doctors for years for recurring infections, allergies and low energy, and they had not solved any of my problems. I finally hit a wall after my second child and prayed to God to help me find a different solution.

I got my answers.

Dear reader,

I discovered there was another, more proactive way to manage health and wellness then following the advice of a traditional doctor. I was so excited by my paradigm shift that I immediately jumped feet first into a Master Herbalist program WHILE my husband was still in medical school.

You can bet we butted heads at first!

But as time went on, we were able to analyze the opposite systems of medicine together, and see that each had its strengths and weaknesses. We were able to see that there were so many proactive things we could do at home before we ever considered going to a conventional doctor.

Since that time, Mike's been practicing medicine as an ER physician and I received a Master Herbalist degree and practice in using the most powerful natural medicine: essential oils, on my family of seven children.

And . . . . I am not alone.

I've found numerous, influential women who have traveled a similar path of discovering a different way to do things.

SO, if you read this book, YOU WILL:

- Discover 25 natural medicine confessions from influential women across the country, and learn which remedies have worked best for each one
- **Find new ways to make your family healthier, and avoid the doctor over and over again**
- Learn easy ways to protect yourself and family from synthetic medicine and it's negative side effects
- **Gain empowering ideas on how to have the confidence to avoid toxic treatments for yourself and loved ones**
- See how women everywhere are choosing more natural therapies that heal themselves and their family members
- **Know how changes in our traditional paradigm can revolutionize your health**

God did help me find amazing solutions for my health (and they weren't from conventional medicine). You can find solutions too.

I promise that if you read all of these stories, you will save a whole lot of money, time and grief. But you have to do your part. By studying and rereading all the experiences in this book, you can learn from others how to take control of your own health and home medicine.

Don't wait to read or buy this book! It will change your paradigm. It will inspire and educate you. If you want to cross the chasm from conventional medicine to natural, follow in the footsteps of those who have already done it. It's worth EVERY PENNY.

I overcame my recurring health issues, reclaimed wellness and the vitality I need because I wanted to raise a large family.

If you don't know how to use natural tools, or even what they are, then you are walking around with a blindfold on, waiting to be shocked by a medical crisis, and once the crisis hits, you often have no choice but to choose conventional medicine at that point.

So, get out your pen and notepad, so you're ready to write down your biggest "aha" gems as you read these power-packed stories and tips for getting started and using more natural remedies for your own medicine and healing!

How Did An MD Husband and Master Herbalist Wife Come To Terms About Medicine?

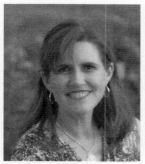

By Jenni Wilson, M.H. http://www.MomEssentials.net, http://www.NaturalMedicineMom.com

I used to bite my nails until my fingers bled. I bit them so low that there was hardly any nail left. I bit them voraciously, and it would cause me to be in pain for days at a time. I've done it for the majority of my life, actually. I used to think it was just a bad habit—that I just needed to keep trying new things to break the habit. I didn't realize there was a powerful imbalance in my body that would continue to manifest itself in many different ways and with many different symptoms.

I ate a lot of sugar growing up. My mother tried to feed us a semi-healthy diet, but I remember hoarding candy, and huge, chocolate chip cookies were a regular standby. I had a little business, making and selling lollipops in junior high school. They were really good, so course I had to eat a lot of them.

Whenever we would get seriously ill, we would go to the doctor and get antibiotics. I did not realize it, but this was wiping out my healthy intestinal flora, and allowing yeast to take over. With all the sugar I ate on top of that, I was feeding the yeast, which just caused me to have more sugar cravings. I was caught in a vicious cycle and developed nervousness, anxiety, and the insatiable addiction to biting my nails.

The problem only got worse when I went to college and my diet was even less healthy. I experienced mood swings and regular illness due to a weak immune system. I started getting urinary tract infections and every winter I would have a severe bout of bronchitis. I had many food allergies and felt like I was always walking a tight rope regarding what I could eat versus what would make me sick.

When I married, I started getting vaginal yeast infections in addition to the UTIs. I would do the standard treatment, but it seemed like a month or two later I would just get another infection. I felt like I was sick all the time with one thing or another. I developed year-round hay fever, with continual runny nose and sneezing. Sometimes I could not stop sneezing for minutes at a time, all day long.

What I didn't realize was that all of these problems were my body's way of showing me that my internal environment was poorly nourished, polluted and imbalanced. I took no thought about the fact that my body might need cleaning on the inside as well as the outside. I knew our diet could be healthier, as it consisted of refined foods and packaged meals. But I had no clue of where to start and what would really make a difference. I just continued to get frustrated with my health until I found myself at such low energy after our second child that I could hardly function.

I had prayed on and off over the years about my health, but I started pleading more fervently than ever. I wanted to have a large family, but I knew it would take much more energy than I had. I was finally ready to make some major lifestyle changes.

One day, after my husband had just started medical school, my sister mentioned that she was going to see a natural doctor. This peaked my interest. I told her I wanted to go too. When we arrived, we had our fingers pricked, and we were showed what our blood and cells looked like on a computer screen. I was fascinated. Some of my cells were spikey, which they said was caused by damage. I also had yeast and other junk floating around in my blood stream. It was the perfect visual aid for grabbing my full attention.

Next, I wanted to know how to get all that junk out of my blood and wondered if it would help me feel better. They assured me that indeed, it would. They proceeded to tell me that I needed to get all the junk out of my diet in order to get the junk out of my blood. That made sense. They began to tell me about salads, vegetables, fruits, whole grains and foods I had never heard of before. I knew I was in for a challenge, but I was ready to take it on! I had a warm peaceful feeling that this was an answer to my prayers, and this path would help be become healthier.

I called my husband on the spot and asked him if he would support me and join me in a real food challenge. Fortunately, he said yes. When I got home, we discarded almost everything in our pantry, and I went to the health food store to do some shopping.

I think we ate brown rice and steamed vegetables for two months straight, but an amazing thing happened. After those two months, all of my allergy symptoms and fatigue disappeared! I started feeling better than I had in years, and wasn't getting sick anymore.

At this point, my interest was piqued by a related topic: natural health and herbal medicine. My sister and mother were so interested that my mom invested, paying up front, for an independent study, Master Herbalist degree through Dr. Christopher's Natural School of Healing for all three of us!

I was so excited, I dove right in, reading as much as I could, filling out the study guides, watching videos and trying remedies on myself and my children. I was amazed that everything I was reading made sense and seemed so reasonable. I wondered why more people didn't know about these "natural remedies," and why our conventional medicine didn't include them in practice.

One day I got into a conversation with Mike, my medical student husband, about how we would be treating our children for fevers in the future. I was reading about Dr. Christopher's Cold Sheet Treatment for fevers and pondering how to do an easy version on kids. Mike was of the opinion that we should take them to the pediatrician or give them an over-the-counter medication. We were soon able to do a test.

It was close to Christmas time and when we were visiting my parents on Christmas Eve, our 4 year-old son came down with a fever. So I gave him Dr. Christopher's Kid-e-Well liquid formula and put him in a hot bath (not burning) to try to get him to sweat (sweat can get lots of infection out of the body). I kept him in there as long as possible, but he didn't really sweat. The next day, Christmas, he had no fever! I was thinking I was awesome!

That night we traveled to the home of Mike's parents, and I left early to do post-holiday shopping. Mike called me on my cell phone and told me that the fever was back, and this time our daughter had it too. He said if I couldn't take care of it, we should take them to a doctor the next day. I felt like this was my big test!

I went home and called the School of Natural Healing to see what I was doing wrong. They said I was doing all the right things, but I needed to do them more. So that night, I put both kids in the bath again, with a tablespoon of ginger powder in the water, had them drink as much juice and peppermint tea (infusion) as they could, and put them in a hot bath for as long as they could stand it. The real danger with fevers is if it's a "dry" fever, meaning the person is not getting enough liquids into the body and gets dehydrated. So drinks are crucial, baths help with hydration, and in a pinch, an enema can be used for hydration if they refuse to drink.

The kids drank, took even more Kid-e-Well, and got hot in the bath. I took them out and put their pajamas directly on without drying them, so they were slightly damp. I put their socks in the water and wrung them out before putting them on, so the moisture would hydrate them all night. Then I put them into a big bed with me, and lots of blankets over us to help them sweat.

It worked! In the morning, both children had broken their fevers and felt much better. This time, the fever didn't come back!

This was a turning point in how we communicated about medicine. I stopped being so pushy about the things I was learning, and Mike started being more positive and letting me try all the things I wanted to do. Over time, we have seen many natural treatments work very well. There have been times when we needed conventional help for stitches, staples and other urgent situations.

I continued the master herbalist program. I worked through levels on and off through babies, moving and home building. I finally finished the program, but it took me 8 years.

A few years before I finished my master herbalist degree, someone introduced me to essential oils. Then a midwife gave me more to use on my last few babies and for various health issues. I was very impressed with how well they worked and how easy they were to use.

When I finished the master herbalist program, I enrolled in an aromatherapy program with the same school. After completing half the work, I lost or misplaced my books. I was so frustrated! I loved what I was learning, still and didn't want to start all over again. I waited for them to turn up. It took almost a year for me to find half of my misplaced materials. By then I had reordered them. As of the publication date of this book, I still have not finished the program. I will at some point. I have since found an excellent certification available for "Aromatic Science and

Essential Oil Application" at http://www.aromaticscience.com/education. I am also exploring ways of validating natural treatments and sharing these remedies with others including health professionals using another exciting online tool, http://www.protocolled.com.

Now when my kids aren't feeling well, I pull out my box of essential oils and rub them down. Here are the ways I've used them just in the couple weeks before writing this:

- My teen daughter had a fever and some digestive upset, so I rubbed some tummy oils on her stomach and bottoms of feet (this is a great place to rub the oils if you don't know where or how else to use them). She felt much better a few hours later.

- My toddler loves to open my essential oils and tap the top with his index finger. Then he rubs that dab of oil on the back of his neck (it's so cute!). So I give him a bottle of a calming blend of essential oils to dab on his neck. This really helps him relax and be ready for sleep.

- I had some semi-serious dental work done, and my dentist was worried that I would be very sore. As soon as I got home, I rubbed some essential oils (including myrrh) on the outside of my cheek. I did this a few times during the day. The discomfort was very minimal. The next morning when I awoke, my jaw was sore on one side. I applied the oils once and the soreness disappeared until the next morning. I repeated using the oils for 3 days, and by then all the soreness and discomfort were completely gone.

- My young daughter came in crying and saying that her leg was hurting. She had not hurt it externally, but said it hurt on the inside. I gave her some essential oils for pain in a lotion to apply to her leg. She took a bath, and afterward was fine.

- My grade school son woke up with a fever, and didn't feel well. I rubbed some immune oils on his feet along with just one drop of peppermint essential oil on the bottom of each foot. He slept for 45 minutes and was back to normal when he woke up.

- My preschool age son is constantly getting bruises and scrapes. We immediately apply essential oils (like lavender, diluted melaleuca, helichrysum or frankincense) to immediately stop bleeding, take down inflammation and diminish or halt the pain. Seriously, the stuff is miraculous!

- Some plans I've made have not gone as smoothly as I expected. When I am feeling stressed, I get out my calming oils and smell them deeply right out of the bottle, or rub them on my neck, along with some orange essential oil. The citruses seem to always help me improve my mood.

These are just some examples of how we use essential oils in our home day to day. But they are powerful enough to reduce disease, fight infection and superbugs, increase longevity, alleviate many different kinds of symptoms, and improve overall wellness.

Natural medicine has definitely changed my life, and I am passionate about sharing life-changing information with others. It's empowering to have natural tools in our homes that we can try first, before seeking for professional (and often expensive) assistance.

I am so excited to introduce you to some fantastic women, who are pioneers in sharing ideas and information about natural health with the world. They become somewhat transparent and vulnerable in the pages of this book, sharing their most personal stories. I know you will be inspired and hopefully motivated by them to think differently and perhaps try something new and empowering in your own life.

About Jenni Wilson, M.H.

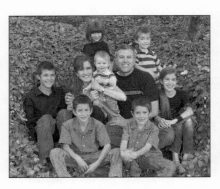

Jenni Wilson, Natural Medicine Mom, is a master herbalist, wife of an ER doctor and mother to 7 children. She teaches women (and a few brave dads) how to use natural tools, and especially essential oils, to care for their families and enjoy more confidence, control and effectiveness in their home health care. She is an author, speaker and natural medicine coach for moms.

Your lifestyle – how you live, eat, and think – determines your health. To prevent disease, you may have to change how you live.

~Brian Carter

Are you new to natural? Katie of Wellness Mama teaches in the next chapter how to get back to basics. She is a mom who discovered first hand how natural remedies can be more effective than conventional medicine at times and how a holistic approach can often bring comfort more quickly. Her natural remedies for ear infection helped her little ones sleep easily and recover more quickly.

Katie from WellnessMama.com found out the hard way that conventional medicine isn't always the best option and turned to natural and holistic remedies when conventional alternatives weren't offering relief or long term healing for her family. Here is her story of her journey to learning natural remedies.

Back to Basics: Using Natural Tools to Heal Colds and Ear Infection

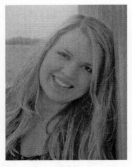

by Katie of WellnessMama.com, http://WellnessMama.com

The journey to healthier eating and natural remedies was a gradual one for me, though it became much more of a priority when I had children.

Prior to having my first child, I didn't really think much about the effect that foods or medicines had on my body. I'd take a pain reliever or decongestant without a second thought and my diet consisted largely of foods I wouldn't even eat now.

My first pregnancy made me realize that everything I was eating or exposed to would now be affecting my child, and I started to research healthy options. I couldn't take most conventional medications during pregnancy and turned to a healthier diet and natural methods (vitamins, herbs, etc) instead.

This eventually led to me going back to school for Nutrition and developing a passion for discovering foods and natural remedies that would promote optimal health, especially for families and small children.

Life with small children often gave me the opportunity to test the effectiveness of safer natural options and until we fully switched to a healthier diet, they sometimes struggled with things like ear infections or colds.

The conventional treatment for these ailments would be antibiotics and fever reducers, but now that I understood the effect these medicines had on the body, I wanted to avoid them unless absolutely necessary and not turn to them for every ear infection or runny nose.

That being said, these minor illnesses can make little ones miserable and can often cause the entire family to lose sleep when the little one has trouble sleeping. I set out to find natural remedies for minor illnesses that would help the child stay more comfortable but that would not interfere with the body's natural healing process.

My studies in nutrition taught me that foods like white flour, sugar and dairy can feed an infection and extend an illness, so at the first sign of illness, we avoided these foods and instead focused on foods like homemade soups and bone broth, cooked vegetables and herbal teas until the afflicted felt better.

As I discovered more about the benefits of using herbs, I also found that herbs and natural remedies could greatly help the symptoms of minor illnesses and encourage the body's natural healing response. For many minor childhood illnesses like cold and earache, medicines like antibiotics are ineffective anyway due to the nature of the illness, and in these cases, natural remedies are even more effective.

I got the chance to test all of my theories when my oldest son picked up a double ear infection and cold (after being on vacation and eating many foods he wouldn't normally have had). When I was a child, these types of illnesses often developed into strep or more serious illness for me and I'd had to have tubes multiple times. I knew the possible severity of illnesses like this, but I also trusted that with support, his body would be able to recover.

Unfortunately, he was very uncomfortable, as can be expected with a double ear infection and cold, so it was tempting to turn to conventional pain relief options just to make him more comfortable. I'd treated some illnesses with only natural medicine before but this was the most severe illness I'd seen in any of my kids, and in the back of my head, I still had some doubt about the effectiveness of natural remedies. He was two years old at the time, so I was able to use a variety of herbs and natural treatments.

I decided to go ahead with a plan to speed his recovery naturally, while still reserving the option to turn to conventional methods if needed. I used a combination of kid-friendly herbs like chamomile, catnip and yarrow, as well as raw honey mixed with cinnamon. I let him rest and watch a movie (a rarity at our house), while constantly giving him herbal teas with cinnamon and honey mixed in. I also gave him Vitamin C in fresh squeezed orange juice and homemade bone broths and soups.

I put warm (but not hot) garlic infused olive oil into his ears and placed chamomile tea bags over his ears every few hours. He took warm baths in Epsom salts and I rubbed peppermint and eucalyptus oil diluted with coconut oil on his feet and chest to help with the cold symptoms.

I noticed several things immediately: He had much more energy and seemed to be in less pain within a few hours of starting these treatments, and the positive effects kept increasing with time rather than wearing off in a few hours. He also slept more soundly with the relief from the natural remedies and was content to read books and watch a movie with me. He broke his fever naturally by that evening and it didn't return.

The most noticeable difference I saw, however, was in the two days following the day we started using natural remedies. He woke up the next morning with close to his normal energy levels and with no complaints of ear pain. Usually, ear infections or colds took several days to kick, at least, and he was almost back to normal by the next day!

The following day, his runny nose was gone, he didn't complain of ear pain and he wanted to eat, drink and play normally.

Since then, I've handled other minor illnesses, infections, and even spider bites at home with natural remedies. As our family's nutrition has continued to improve, we don't get sick as often, but herbs and natural remedies have been helpful in cases of small cuts or infections and even in cases of more major problems like food poisoning. The same treatments I used on my son for his ear infections and colds have also been effective for my husband and I and for our other children (though some were diluted for small children).

Tips and Tricks from Along the Way

From my experience with using natural remedies to help speed recovery from illnesses like colds, ear ache and even the flu, I've picked up some tricks along the way. I am now a firm believer in the effectiveness of natural remedies since with four children, we haven't had to visit a doctor to treat an illness or injury in over five years (since we started using natural remedies).

Unlike conventional medicine, natural remedies do take some advance preparation. A prescription for antibiotics is pretty easy to get last minute when an illness strikes, but unusual or out of season herbs or remedies that take weeks to prepare can't easily be made once an illness strikes. I now keep an "herbal medicine chest" in a cabinet in our kitchen so that if an illness strikes I am prepared to handle it.

The most important thing I've realized with using natural remedies is that it is important to realize that in most cases (and there are certainly exceptions), the human body, and especially a child's body, is designed to heal and overcome illness. When we support the body's natural response with methods that assist the natural healing process, natural remedies can be both more effective and faster than many conventional methods. Overcoming small illnesses without the help of conventional medicines is actually good for the body and for immune system development, and as a parent, I have to trust this natural process rather than turning to medicine at the first sign of any issue.

It can certainly be very difficult to watch a child suffer, even mildly, from an illness, but I've found that natural remedies can speed the process and help the child maintain comfort during the healing time.

One remedy that we use often for everything from teething pain to ear infection is homemade **Chamomile Tincture**. Here's the very easy recipe, and this and other tincture recipes are available on WellnessMama. com:

Ingredients

- 3/4 cup dried chamomile flowers
- Enough boiling distilled water to cover flowers (about a cup)
- 2 cups of vodka or rum
- a Quart size mason jar with tight fitting lid

Instructions

Place the chamomile flowers in the glass jar and pour boiling distilled water over the chamomile just to wet all of the flowers (the heat helps release compounds in the chamomile)

Fill the rest of the jar with vodka or rum and put on the lid.

Store in a cool, dark place for 4-6 weeks, shaking the jar daily. The beneficial properties of the chamomile will infuse into the liquid to create a tincture with an indefinite shelf life.

After 4-6 weeks, strain the flowers out using several layers of cheesecloth and store the tincture in jars or small tincture bottles.

To Use

We use the finished tincture directly on the gums for teething children and on the stomach or head externally on small babies and children for colic and tummy troubles.

For older children, I dilute 15 drops in a small glass of water and set out for 15 minutes so that the alcohol can evaporate and then give to the child to drink. I use this dose every few hours to help with pain and symptoms until illness is gone.

For adults, up to 40 drops can be used as needed. Chamomile's relaxing properties also make this a helpful bedtime aid for children who are having trouble sleeping.

Other methods I use to help with minor illnesses:

- For children older than 1 year and adults, I mix 1/4 tsp cinnamon into a teaspoon of honey and give directly or mix into herbal tea.
- For ear pain, I use hydrogen peroxide in the ear at first sign of discomfort and then use warm (not hot) olive oil with garlic infused in it to help the body fight the infection.
- During illness, we drink an abundance of water and herbal teas including chamomile, catnip, yarrow, peppermint and nettle (or a mixture of all of those)
- Homemade elderberry syrup has also been helpful, especially for cold and flu.
- Warm Epsom salt baths help the natural detoxification and healing reactions of the body and also provide relaxation and comfort (as well as a good boost of magnesium).
- Homemade bone broth/stock and soups made from homemade broths provide minerals and gelatin to aid the body in the healing process. I often make a big batch of homemade chicken soup at the first sign of illness.
- Avoiding all "white" foods like flour, sugar and dairy can often speed illness recovery.
- Vitamin C powder mixed into freshly squeezed orange juice provides an immune boost and kids often enjoy drinking it.
- Maintaining good gut bacteria with fermented foods and probiotics will help avoid illness, and will also help speed recovery.

- Essential oils like peppermint and eucalyptus can help sooth coughing and congestion with diluted in a carrier oil like olive or coconut and rubbed on feet or chest (not for use in very small babies).
- For babies and small children, nursing provides the best protection against illness and exclusively nursing children under 1 during an illness will often help speed the recovery process.

There are certainly times when conventional medicine is needed, and I'm very grateful that it is available at these times, but in many cases, natural remedies will not only be more effective but better for the body in the long term since they aid the healing response rather than just mask symptoms or take over the job of the immune system.

Natural remedies can often offer not only a comparable, but a better alternative to conventional treatments for minor ailments. I hope that my experience will encourage you to do your own research into the world of natural remedies.

About Katie

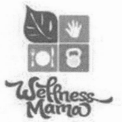

Katie of *Wellness Mama is a full-time housewife with a background in nutrition, journalism and communications. Her passion is helping others achieve optimal health through a "Wellness Lifestyle." She has helped clients lose weight, increase athletic performance, improve fertility, and more.*

When she's not working or blogging, she's spending time with her family, watching movies, reading fantasy novels, listening to opera, and beating her former classmates at Scramble with Friends. She is very grateful for the opportunity to be included in this book.

Surgeons must be very careful
When they take the knife!
Underneath their fine incisions
Stirs the culprit-Life!

~Emily Dickenson

Natural medicine is not just a trend to try. Read in the next chapter how switching to natural medicine may have saved Patty's life. It is an amazing story that illustrates why conventional medicine is not always a "sure thing." Don't miss Patty of "Loving Our Guts" who shares her easiest recipe for helping you find relief for colds and illness. Learn from her clear view of the differences between natural and conventional medicine.

When I first heard Patty's story, I was crushed inside at the amount of suffering she had to endure while learning the risks and hazards of conventional medicine and surgery. It's eye opening! You definitely need to read on as she gives powerful evidence of why we should consider alternatives to invasive treatments, and what can happen if we don't.

Conventional Medicine Left Me Helpless

by Patty Lacoss-Arnold, http://www.lovingourguts.com

In the past I've practiced a combination of conventional and alternative approaches to health. Growing up we used a combination of both when we were got ill. When we got colds, my parents encouraged us to take lots of vitamin C and to drink hot honey lemonade.

My father was always interested in natural cures and when they learned that I was progressing toward a need for glasses, he started the whole family on daily cod liver oil. Well not only did it prevent my needing glasses (I still don't wear them and am over 40), but my father's eyesight actually improved significantly and he was no longer considered legally blind without his glasses!

In my 20's I discovered that taking cod liver oil and drinking red raspberry tea greatly diminished my pains with my cycle, so I never went without them again. However, with sinus infections or similar illness, I quickly went to the doctor to get antibiotics. There was no doubt in my mind that they were necessary for those illnesses. I also eagerly lined up for extra vaccinations if they were suggested for any reason. Back then, in my mind, conventional medicine was the sure thing and while I preferred to start with natural approaches I did not hesitate to switch to a more conventional treatment if my first attempts didn't seem to be working fast enough.

At that time in my life, I did not have a very well thought-out philosophy on why I used natural medicine first with illness. Mostly, I think it just seemed like something to try that might help and it was less expensive and time consuming than a trip to the doctor. Plus I knew that there was little for a doctor to do for the "common cold" or a virus. Taking some vitamin c and drinking hot lemon tea helped me to feel like I was doing something. I never really expected it to have a significant impact on the length of my cold, although it would help with its severity. If I had an illness that I thought a doctor could help with, I did not hesitate to make an appointment. After all . . . who wants to stay sick?

Shortly after I got married I learned that my monthly menstrual pain was not normal and might be indicative of Endometriosis. My sister and close friend experienced worse pain than I did, so I had assumed it was a normal part of life for most women. Once the problem had a name I began to research as much as I could about this disease. I quickly became convinced that a specific technique to remove this overgrowth was the best approach.

My next step was to seek out a local doctor who was trained in this specialized kind of surgery. I found one and immediately liked her a lot. She seemed to share my views that natural and conventional medicine could be combined to achieve health. She had studied with "the top" Endometriosis surgeon, learned his techniques, and was highly regarded among the medical community as being a great surgeon in her own right. I quickly scheduled surgery with her in hopes that I would soon be feeling much better.

My first sign that things were not going as planned was when I woke up from surgery. I was told that instead of going home that day as I expected, I was going to be spending the night in the hospital on a morphine pump. Apparently, I had not recovered well from the extensive surgery and she did not want to send me home until I was more stable. I went home from the hospital and planned to spend a week recuperating before I returned to work.

After a week I was still needing painkillers all the time. I attempted to return to work, but after one day back it was clear that I wasn't able to do my job and I took a leave of absence. My doctor ran some tests and decided that the continued pain meant I had an infection at the surgery site. When I couldn't tolerate the oral antibiotics she gave me, she prescribed 2 weeks of IV antibiotics. (Can you see how quickly this is escalating?)

Once the antibiotics were done, I still was in pain but showing no signs of infection. My doctor did not know why, or how to help me, but she kept writing me scripts for my painkillers. I went to my internist and got a physical hoping she would find a cause for my pain and she pronounced me perfectly healthy.

I went to see another surgeon for a second opinion about my condition. He had no idea what was wrong either. I struggled to walk because of my pain and weakness. I used wheelchairs or motorized carts when I went to stores or anywhere out in public that required much walking. I did not drive for months because I was always on painkillers and did not dare get behind the wheel of a car. Worst of all, when I got my period, the pain was more excruciating than ever. I even fainted from the pain of it one month and woke up on the floor of my bathroom.

Finally, I had exhausted all the conventional medical approaches and I began to ask friends who were more natural minded if they knew anyone that might help me. Thankfully, the first referral I got was to a brilliant chiropractor who quickly devised a plan to help me. He also happened to know my surgeon and had a high opinion of her. This doctor prescribed a homeopathic remedy for my pain that immediately got me off the painkillers that I was living on. I had seriously underestimated the power of alternative medicine! I never imagined it could work better than the prescription narcotics that I was taking.

Soon, I was growing stronger and began to drive again but I still did not feel well enough to return to work or walk much in public. While I was visiting my parents out of state, my mother insisted that I should go to see her massage therapist who was experienced in Cranial Sacral Therapy (CST). That kind woman worked on me for nearly 2 hours, which was much longer than a typical session. It is difficult to describe all that I experienced in that session with her. After she worked on me, I was convinced that this was a key to my further healing so I found a local chiropractor who was experienced in CST.

At my first appointment with this new chiropractor, she got me standing up straight for the first time since before my surgery. I hadn't even realized how hunched over I was until I was standing up straight again.

Soon, I was able to contact my boss and say that I was ready to return to work. I was still weak and needed to be careful to not overdo it, but what a victory that I could work again! I had begun to wonder if I was going to be using a wheelchair for the rest of my life. Indeed, if I had listened exclusively to the conventional doctors, I might have been. They had no answers for me other than to wait and take prescription painkillers. It was the alternative practitioners that I met who had healing options to offer me.

That experience was a real turning point in my life. While I tended to reach for "alternative" medicine first much of the time, I usually sought out the "big guns" of conventional medicine for anything that didn't respond quickly and seemed to be turning into a "significant" problem. I thought of conventional medicine as the "sure thing" and other approaches as weak and uncertain. I never really considered that conventional medicine could have a significant down side to it. Those side effects and risks seemed to be for other people, until they happened to me.

Conventional medicine pronounced me "perfectly healthy" while I could barely function day to day. That really opened my eyes to the limits to the standard of care here in America. As long as the lab tests came back in range, there was nothing wrong with me. I knew differently, but I needed to find some new practitioners to get some answers and regain my life.

Once that paradigm had shifted, there was a whole new world that opened up for me. That first chiropractor who got me off painkillers, also introduced me to the concept of diet influencing health beyond weight management. What an amazing new world of ideas that opened up to me! Now I often forget that most people do not think this way about food. It is my firmly held belief that any pursuit of health that does not address diet in a significant way is ultimately doomed to fail.

This idea of food being the foundation to health shifted the power to heal into my realm. In my house I am the grocery shopper and meal maker for my family. It is my understanding of diet that will heal or harm us. I had to learn which foods were best for each of us and then seek to balance our diets around those principles. What a responsibility! What power!

When I began to change our diets, I could see that indeed it had great influence on us in many more ways than we ever imagined. The foods that we ate influenced our moods, wellbeing, sleep, and body shapes, sometimes quite dramatically. I often think back to when we first tried a grain free diet. Despite the extra work in the kitchen, after about a month, my marriage was much happier. Clearly the foods we had been eating were affecting us negatively in subtle ways that we could not recognize until they were removed from our diet.

Once I fully understood my power to heal through nutrition, I was empowered to learn more. Moving on to understanding herbs, essential oils, homeopathic remedies and other "alternative" approaches was the next logical step. Rushing to the doctor when my child has a weird rash or a sore throat is not the way that we handle things any more. Instead I rush to my books and remedies and address the problem quickly at home. My doctor is there if an issue is beyond my skills but the more I learn and the more experience I gain, the less we need her help with acute illnesses.

Now, when my gallbladder acts up I apply a couple of drops of an essential oil blend over the area and the pain quickly goes away. When I saw a doctor about my gall bladder pain he offered to remove it surgically and wrote me a prescription for a heavy-duty painkiller. Neither of those approaches would heal my gall bladder. They would simply stop the pain and come with their own side effects. The essential oils stop the pain without any side effects. Did you know that people without gall bladders are at risk of getting deficient in the fat-soluble vitamins because their digestion does not effectively digest fats any longer in the absence this organ? Keeping my gall bladder and working to heal it means that I will continue to be able to digest fats and maintain my stores of fat-soluble vitamins.

Conventional medicine often just manages symptoms. At times that is very welcome, but other times it stops people from looking for real answers and healing of the cause since the symptoms are managed. In some cases, the conventional medical treatment may fix one problem just to create other symptoms that must also be treated. Alternative medicine often has ways to support healing—not just management of symptoms—and I love that!

Also, approximately 100,000 Americans die each year from side effects of medicine that they took according to the instructions. Zero people die most years from taking herbs according to directions. Which is not to say that they are powerless placebos. They simply have a greater safety margin and minimal side effects when used according to accepted practices.

In conclusion, I would like to share one of my favorite remedies for any sort of infection in the body. This seems to work best if you use it at the first sign of illness and thankfully contains ingredients that most people have on hand in their house or can easily get if necessary. I have used this to fight off infections of all kinds including mastitis that was causing a high fever. This remedy has been shared with my family and friends and many of them now use it as well.

Apple Cider Vinegar in Juice

Simply add 1-2 tbsp of apple cider vinegar to 16 oz of juice and drink it down. Many a skeptic who was ill and wanting relief has tried this and been convinced of its power. For some it seems to work almost instantly and for others it takes several doses over a couple of days to really find relief.

My family has found much health and healing from incorporating what some call "alternative" medicine into our lives. I encourage you to look into the various approaches out there and find ones that work for your family.

Patty's story shows that alternative medicine has answers that conventional medicine can't touch. It also shows that help from a qualified alternative health care practitioner can mean the difference between a life of pain and medications and vibrant healthy life. While surgery removed her endometriosis, the presumed cause of her pain, it did nothing to improve her quality of life and in fact made it much worse. Thankfully, there are other answers available when conventional doctors don't have them. Even to questions that seem too big for unconventional approaches. It just requires looking in new places.

About Patty Lacoss-Arnold

Patty, a homeschooling mother of two girls, loves singing, cooking and reading a good classic novel. She passionately pursues healthy eating and natural medicine to heal herself and her family. Her family began their healing journey with the GAPS™ diet in November of 2009 but her pursuit of health using holistic methods started long before that. In November of 2011 Patty decided to share with others what she was learning and began her blog "Loving Our Guts." Her blog includes recipes, health information, and personal stories about herself and her family.

As for butter versus margarine,
I trust cows more than chemists.

~Joan Gussow

Don't miss the next chapter, where Kate Tietje demonstrates how eating real food can help lose real weight safely! Learn how her family, a family who had severe allergies, was overweight, and could not solve their health issues despite meeting many doctors, overcame their obstacles when they found real food and natural health!

It's True! We Lost Fat by Eating MORE Fat!

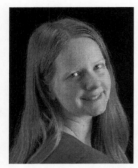

By Kate Tietje, http://www.modernalternativemama.com

This is a story about my dear husband, Ben, and partially written by him (he's driving as we write so I'm "helping" him, haha). Recently, he traveled for business and was forced to eat out for a three and a half days. It inspired us to write "his story" in detail, because it served as a strong reminder to us about why we eat the way we do.

When we met, Ben was working as a retail manager, a job that kept him on his feet most of the day. He usually went out to eat or brought a frozen meal to work. At that point he weighed about 220 lbs. (he is 6'2"). He worked second shift—about 1 PM to 10 PM, five days a week. He typically skipped breakfast, ate frozen food for lunch, and when he got home, had fast food. He didn't have time to prepare anything that wasn't premade. Even on his days off, he usually ate this way, with the rare exceptions of making spaghetti or chili (but used prepared/canned ingredients and white pasta).

When we got married in 2006, Ben left his job as a retail manager and began a new job sitting at a desk all day. He gained some weight, topping out at 235 lbs. in the summer of 2007. At this time, we ate "better" but by no means well. When we got married a typical meal in our house was Rice'a'roni and baked chicken, or soup made with canned broth, conventional veggies, and factory-farmed chicken breast. We never felt well. Every night after dinner we just sat around feeling terrible.

Neither of us could understand why we were gaining weight when we were eating "well" by SAD (Standard American Diet) standards. We went out to eat once or twice a week, made boxed or frozen foods, but also cooked some for ourselves. We ate a low-fat diet as much as possible, focusing on boneless, skinless chicken, frozen veggies, margarine, vegetable oil, etc. Yet our weight continued to climb. I topped out at 143, which is when I got pregnant with my first child. I weighed 170 lbs. when I was 9 months pregnant.

In late 2007, in an effort to combat our weight gain, Ben started to work out. He ran several mornings a week and also worked with weights. He did this for several months with no effect on his weight. Then, he was very sore and having back problems and quit. In March 2008, Ben started an exercise program again. By this time we were slowly starting to change our diet. We were still not eating or feeling very well while eating a low-fat diet, and though Ben was running on a treadmill for about 2 miles almost every day, there was still no effect on his weight.

Towards the end of 2008, when I got pregnant again, we found the Weston A. Price Foundation and started to read about higher fat diets and different food choices. We began to incorporate some of these principles in our diet and began to lose weight. I was down to 127 lbs. before I got pregnant with our second. Ben began to lose weight, too. He got down to around 210 by early 2009, when we got a Wii with Wii Fit. Daily cardio on the Wii accelerated his weight loss a little bit, although we only did it for about a month. I was about 6 months pregnant and gaining weight slowly.

It was towards the end of my second pregnancy that we really started to focus on fats. We bought coconut oil and I made smoothies everyday with a lot of coconut oil. We baked fries in coconut or olive oil. We began to eat a lot of real butter. We ate a TON of food and a lot of fat and our weight began to drop. By the end of 2009, I weighed around 125 lbs. and Ben weighed around 190 lbs.

In early 2010 we focused even more heavily on meat and fat. We'd gotten grass-fed beef at the end of 2009 and ate a lot of that, a lot of coconut oil, lots of coconut milk, olive oil, whatever we could find that was high in fat. We cut out grains entirely in January 2010 for about two months, as well as sugar. During this time our weight fell further, Ben's reaching down to 175 lbs. and mine to 113 lbs. at our lowest. Ben's weight has remained stable there, mine rose to about 118 lbs. after I began eating grains again (but I suspect that at my height, 5'3", and frame, that 113 was a bit too low).

Ben was at 175 lbs. when he left on a trip recently. While he was gone, he ate as well as he could—meat, dairy, fruits and vegetables, minimal grains. He did not have the option to choose raw dairy, grass-fed meat, or organic produce however. When he came home, despite eating less than usual, and not choosing "horrible" choices (i.e. fried foods, high sugar foods), he had gained 5 lbs. He also had gotten a cold and felt very fatigued and generally ill. It took him only three days eating real food again to lose the weight, and within a few days he felt much better.

When we choose whole, real foods with plenty of real fat and minimal grains (choosing sprouted whole grains when we do have them), our weight remains low naturally, no matter how much we eat. We eat until we are satisfied, which is different on different days. We generally feel quite good all the time, rarely getting sick and having plenty of energy.

Also, as we've mentioned before, Ben had lost some of his hair and it wasn't growing back. At its worst, his hair completely stopped growing for over two months. When we began to eat more fat, and stopped using our microwave to heat food (and never, ever in plastic, even when traveling), his hair began to grow back—after over a year and a half! All of the signs of health began to return when we ate healthy, whole foods. Our kids don't ever burn in the sun, even after 2+ hours of direct exposure with no sunscreen at all. I burn, but only on my back/shoulders or other areas that don't often get exposed. I used to burn everywhere, badly, but my legs, arms, neck and face no longer burn. I have watched plump little children playing in the sun, slathered in SPF 45, still burning. These are ominous signs of a lack of health.

Our modern diet is not healthy. Conventionally grown produce, corn-fed animals, microwaves, food stored in plastics, foods that are packaged and processed, chemical food ingredients, etc. are causing a myriad of problems which may or may not seem obvious, but which are affecting our health in both the short—and long—term.

Unfortunately most people lump sugar and fat in the same category as bad, to be avoided at all costs. Fat is good for you! White sugar is bad. Remember that.

Now, I love natural remedies. **I love knowing that I can treat most of the acute illnesses that crop up in my family at home, without need of a doctor or any prescriptions.** In my opinion, *that* is how it should be! We save doctors and drugs for serious times (and if you think a situation occurring in your home *is* serious, please don't hesitate to seek a doctor's opinion).

But I know that even though I've built up quite a bit of knowledge on what works for various symptoms, I am often at a loss when illness actually strikes. I have remedies on hand . . . but sometimes not exactly the right stuff, or sometimes what I have on hand isn't "prepared" properly. When you have anti-nausea herbs around but no tinctures or even teas ready to go, and someone says "I need something *now* or I'm going to throw up," well . . . you're caught off guard. That's no good!

Why Create a Homemade Medicine Kit?

I have four small children. Life with them is *busy*. And they get hurt. They get sick (sometimes). Mostly, they bounce back in minutes to hours. Sometimes they experience pain. The vast majority of these little bumps and sniffles don't require any sort of doctor's care, but I don't want to just leave my kids in pain, either.

There are many over-the-counter (OTC) remedies around, but I don't consider most of these safe. We don't even own ibuprofen. Children's cold and cough medicine is no longer approved for children under 6 (and in my opinion, really shouldn't be taken at all). I don't usually consider OTC options when I'm looking for something to help my children or myself, or my husband, feel better.

There are also many homeopathic and herbal preparations available out there, and they are (usually) safe. However, they are expensive. Each little blue tube of homeopathic remedy costs $7 or so, and although it lasts for quite awhile—you really need several different ones. A tube or tin of ointment could cost $10+. You get the picture—**buying all the prepared remedies you need costs a lot of money**. Plus, you're limited to what's available in your area, or what can be ordered on the internet, and the remedy that would work best for your family may or may not even be available!

(For example—my cough and cold syrup has been super effective for my family. I can't say that buying a store-bought natural type would have worked so well, and it certainly would have cost more. I've never seen anything on the market that is very close to my homemade version.)

Homemade remedies are cheaper, safer (as long as you're careful), and customizable!

In the span of 5 years, our family overcame being overweight, severe food allergies, speech delays, heavy metal toxicity, and more. All of this was possible with our move towards healthier food and homemade medicine, even after doctor after doctor failed us.

About Kate Tietje

Kate Tietje is wife to Ben and mommy to four. She is passionate about God, health, and food. She is the founder of ModernAlternativeMama. com and has several popular pages on Facebook. She has written many information packed, healthy cookbooks. When she's not blogging, she's in the kitchen, sewing, or homeschooling her children. She loves empowering women in greater spirituality and health.

Physicians and politicians resemble one another in this respect, that some defend the constitution and others destroy it.

~Author Unknown

Coming up . . . Penny Williams give an excellent overview of natural tools for ADHD! An essay by a mom whose only choice for learning how to parent her son with ADHD, Sensory Processing Disorder, and learning disabilities is through trial by fire. Her journey to helping him achieve a happy and successful life has its highs and lows. She eventually realizes that treatment through a combination of Western medicine and natural practices provides the best results for her little boy.

Addressing ADHD with Alternatives

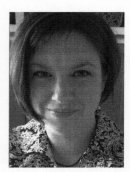

by Penny Williams, http://www.ADHDmomma.com

Raising children is hard. Anyone who disputes that fact doesn't have a child.

Raising a child with neurological differences is exponentially more difficult. The old proverb is true—it does take a village to raise a child, especially when that child has special needs. Ideally, your village includes a combination of traditional and alternative remedies. It can be one harrowing journey to find just the right balance—to build just the right team to care for a child with disabilities—but it is so rewarding to see your child thrive in the end.

My son, Ricochet, is now ten years old. In November 2008, just after his sixth birthday and the start of first grade, he was diagnosed with ADHD. Each year since then, his disability profile has revealed itself to be more complex as general expectations grow greater with age and his ability to meet those expectations falls further and further behind. In second grade, Sensory Processing Disorder (SPD) was added to his list of diagnoses. Dysgraphia & Written Expression Disorder—a deficiency in the ability to write in terms of handwriting and coherence, a writing disorder associated with impaired handwriting, orthographic coding, written expression, and finger sequencing—was added in third grade when his writing still looked like it was produced by a four-year-old, if he could even get any thoughts on paper at all.

With fourth grade came an overwhelming realization that his Executive Functioning Skills were extremely deficient, that revelation is part of the reason he is in fourth grade for the second time this year. But his Gifted Intelligence was one label that never came as a surprise—we recognized his astonishing intelligence at a very young age.

Juggling all these diagnoses and special needs is a challenge at best. The Behavioral M.D. we saw for Ricochet's evaluation and diagnosis immediately prescribed stimulant medication to manage the ADHD symptoms. He said, "You, his parents and his teacher, have already been implementing behavior modification strategies for some time without marked improvement. This is the first-line treatment for ADHD so we can tell he already needs more intervention."

Daddy and I were devastated. We took time to think it over, time to mourn the loss of a "normal" childhood for our son, and then we accepted the prescription and began pharmaceutical treatment of Ricochet's ADHD.

Ricochet did pretty well with the medication. We saw a drastic improvement in his ability to attend in school and even in his writing. But these improvements were always short-lived. Every couple months his dosage was being increased or we were changing the medication altogether. Each new dose or medication began failing in that same short time period. The Behavioral M.D. told me we'd just have to accept that this was as good as it would get for our son. I would not accept that, especially not after seeing glimpses of his potential greatness.

We quickly moved Ricochet's care to a local Behavioral Health practice and, after a year or so, found ourselves giving him the highest dosage of stimulant allowed and trading our smart, sweet, funny little boy for sustained attention in school. This was not a trade we were willing to make. With this realization, we lowered the medication to what we considered a reasonable dosage and took a step back to re-evaluate our son's treatment.

He had been seeing an Occupational Therapist once a week and she helped us develop strategies to cope with his sensory issues and to better understand the whys behind his behaviors. She also worked with him intensely on his handwriting, but with no lasting effect.

This type of therapy helped quite a bit, so what other similar treatments could we discover? What else can we do to possibly augment the efficacy of medication?

I was learning that artificial colors, flavors, and preservatives were not only bad for all of us, but could be exacerbating Ricochet's unwanted behaviors. With this knowledge, we removed as much of these chemicals from his diet as possible, a difficult task after eight years of eating just about anything he wanted. Luke and I began seeing a Pediatric Therapist a couple times a month too—again, facilitating understanding and offering strategies to modify behaviors and improve lagging skills.

About two and a half years after the initial diagnosis, we were able to get health insurance for our children that would cover a doctor practicing Integrative Medicine at the behavioral health practice now responsible for the treatment of Ricochet's ADHD. The volume and cost of the testing she recommended was overwhelming, but we dove in with one test at a time to see what else we could discover about our sweet little boy. We started with IgG food allergy and sensitivity testing.

I was terrified of the results of this particular test. I knew that many children with ADHD also had gluten and/or casein sensitivities and I did not want to take on the daunting task of managing the restrictive diet these sensitivities would require. Of course, they revealed that my child has a gluten sensitivity—he's not sensitive enough to be sick from ingesting gluten, but my research told me this food issue untreated could be wreaking havoc on the efficacy of his medication. I was certain the removal of gluten from Ricochet's diet was going to be the answer we were seeking.

I've learned to not be prematurely sure of anything anymore.

While the removal of gluten from his diet resolved a soiling issue we had battled for more than five years, it did not improve his ADHD behaviors and it did not improve the efficacy of his medication—a success and a failure all in one.

Next we tested for heavy metals toxicity through both hair and urine testing. Both tests showed that he hadn't reached toxicity but there was definitely way too much lead and mercury stored in his tissues. We started right away on oral chelation under the care of Ricochet's Integrative Meds doctor. He takes one DSMA capsule weekly. He is still taking this alternative medication after five or more months. In this time we have seen a great many positive changes in his behavior and maturity. Can I say for sure the improvements are due to the DSMA? No, not at all. There have been many changes in his life since starting DSMA that may have contributed to his growth as well—we moved, changing school districts to one better suited to manage his special needs; he has a much more understanding teacher than last school year; he is repeating the fourth grade to be more closely matched to his peers in maturity and accountability; he is able to go outside in the yard and play whenever he wants in our new home; he is growing up in general; and we finally found a medication balance that is truly effective to manage his ADHD.

Also during our time under the care of the Integrative Meds doctor, we added many vitamin and mineral supplements based on test results. Oddly, there were many supplements Ricochet tested very low on that he simply couldn't tolerate. For instance, a standard dose of B6 or B12 would cause significant aggression and anger, despite being deficient in both. Calcium supplements had the same effect as well. There are certainly still some unsolved mysteries to the chemistry of this amazing little boy.

And the rest of the mysteries will just have to wait. We lost the kids' insurance that covered visits to this alternative doctor and all his mental health caregivers. We now pay out of pocket for every visit to his Behavioral Health Pediatrician and Counselor, so there's no way we could also pay out of pocket in full for a third caregiver.

For our family it has been most important to be open to all sorts of treatments for Ricochet's ADHD and other conditions, accepting treatment recommendations from both traditional Western medicine and alternative medicine as possibilities to help our son create a happy and successful life, in spite of differences.

- Traditional medicine provides pharmaceuticals to help the faulty chemical processes in his brain. Finding the right medication for Ricochet was no easy journey in and of itself. It took three years of trial and error and finally one last Hail-Mary move to discover the medications that are effective in treating his ADHD, without negative complications. After countless stimulants failed after two months of efficacy, his Behavioral Pediatrician prescribed Amantadine—a little-known medication once used for influenza 50 years ago and for Parkinson's Disease today—and it has kept his stimulant working for a year now, and at a much lower dose than without the added medication. This traditional medicine and a little out-of-the-box thinking is essential for Ricochet to achieve academic success.

- Counseling and occupational therapy have offered understanding and acceptance of Ricochet's neurological profile and how we should interact with him in various situations each day for the best possible behavioral outcomes. For instance, we learned that big bear hugs we call a Big Squeeze, with his arms and legs folded in too, could diffuse a situation before it reached full-blown meltdown, a benefit we'd never get in a pill. His therapist has imparted too much insight for me to begin to list here but I am certainly a far better parent of a kid with ADHD and learning disabilities than I'd be without her. She has also helped Ricochet to think through and create a plan to deal with certain situations he struggles with. All invaluable and all things we couldn't achieve through pharmaceutical treatment alone.

- Alternative medicine has proven that there's a big picture to health. We must consider diet as an effective opportunity for transformation and an individual's chemical profile for signs of weakness as well. Many of our bodies' systems interact, and ignoring that fact could cost you effective treatment.

There is so much more to health than Western medicine and first-line treatments alone provide. An open mind and considering all options, traditional or not, has been the saving grace for Riccochet . . . and for our family.

Penny has had quite a journey searching for the best treatment for her son's ADHD, Sensory Processing Disorder and learning disabilities. She learned over time and through many trials that the best treatment for Ricochet is parents with an open mind and a combination of Western and alternative medicine. It is important in parenting and for all of our health to be open to the many ideas for treatment that exist and to cultivate a treatment plan that works for each individual's needs.

About Penny Williams

Penny is the original creator of A Mom's View of ADHD. She is also a freelance writer, real estate broker, wife, and mother of two living in Asheville, N.C. She has published several pieces in ADDitude Magazine, the #1 national publication dedicated to ADHD, and has also been quoted in Parenting.com's Family Health Guide on ADHD and The High Desert Pulse article, When Ritalin Works. When not writing, she can usually be found behind a camera

I saw a few die of hunger—
of eating, a hundred thousand.

~Benjamin Franklin

Whether you are currently sick or not, be sure to read the next chapter, and learn from Brandie Schwartz how to "eat your medicine and eat yourself to LIFE! The information that you can glean from Brandi can help you and your loved ones live healthier lives. In some cases, it may actually save them! You will experience the power of eating real food from the perspective of two people. One is a man who suffered from chronic health conditions. The other is his wife who fought to battle the potentially fatal conditions from which her husband suffered. You will see how eating whole foods changed their lives.

How We Went From Morbidly Obese to Making Changes That Saved My Husband's Life

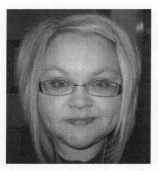

by Brandie Schwartz, CHHC, AADP, RNWCON,
http://EatYourselfToLife.com

Thousands of years ago, Hippocrates, the father of Western medicine, said, "Let thy food be thy medicine, and let thy medicine be thy food." In this short and simple statement, one of the most prominent figures in the history of medicine gave us a small, but important, insight into the manner in which we should attain and maintain our health. Before you reach for a pill or go to the doctor for a shot, try what God intended for us to do. Eat your medicine. Yes, one can eat one's self to life!

Do not misconstrue what I say. Western medicine has a very valid place in the process of maintaining health. In particular, modern western medicine is remarkable in its diagnostic capabilities. It is this very strength that led me down the path of holistic health.

Most of my life has been dedicated to the health and care of others. As a teenager, I volunteered at the local hospital in my hometown, Odessa, Texas. I pursued a nursing career and eventually earned a Registered Nurse's license and a Bachelor's Degree in Nursing. For over 16 years, I watched a cornucopia of humanity pass through the hospital doors. Some had traumatic injuries due to accidents. Others had chronic conditions that more often than not led to tragic ends. I specialized in wound care and ostomy. I noted that patients that maintained a healthy diet healed quicker and more thoroughly than their counterparts that did not have comparably healthy diets.

This fascinated me. My interest in holistic medicine began to captivate me. Additionally, I thanked God that I did not have to deal with the pain of prolonged misery due to disease. However, God has His agenda and I have mine. What was to happen to me next was certainly not part of my agenda.

In 2008, my husband, Bear, and I were faced with one of our greatest fears. My husband was getting a head-to-toe physical to determine his eligibility for a job. As previously stated, this is a major strength of modern Western medicine. The tests he undertook included echocardiograms, A1C, urinalysis, and many more. A couple of the tests came back with results that were a bit disconcerting. His A1C, a test that measures a three-month running average of one's blood sugar, was dangerously high, measuring at 8.7. His urinalysis showed an unusually high amount of protein being spilled in his urine. Ultimately, the diagnosis came back that he was a Type II diabetic and suffering from Chronic Kidney Disease. It was a matter of time before his kidneys would stop functioning all together. My mission was clear. I had to find a way to heal my husband.

While the doctor's began writing prescriptions (over 12) that my husband had to begin taking, I began to do my own research. The diabetes didn't seem to be too much of a problem. Don't eat anything white and stay away from sugar and get some physical activity. So, it would seem, that if my husband wanted something sweet, artificial sweeteners were to be used. However, I began to research what artificial sweeteners would be the best to use. I found that none of them were fit for human consumption. They are not food. They are chemicals . . . and dangerous ones at that! I began to research more substitute foods like margarine and non-dairy creamers. Without exception, I found that these substitute foods were far more dangerous to the consumer than the foods they replaced.

The problem of what to feed my husband loomed in my mind. For years, I had been taught to stay away from sugar, use non-fat or low-fat dairy products, limit meats, eat more fruits and vegetables, and eat whole grains. In part, this model was starting to fall apart. If sugar was bad and sugar substitutes were bad, what would we eat? Slowly, with more and more research, the answers came to me. Simply put, eating real whole food was the answer. This revelation beckoned me to learn more. As a result, I attended the Institute for Integrative Nutrition and started Eat Your Medicine. My husband would be my first client. The results of our hard work would determine the course our future would take.

Before I continue on my husband's improved health, allow me to further explain my husband's health at the beginning of our journey. Bear has always been a large man. At one point in his life, he began having issues with gout. This is a terribly painful form of arthritis that presents itself with uric acid crystals pooling in the joints, usually in the big toe, but sometimes in the ankle, knee, or elbow. Additionally, he had herniated a disc in his back. While these injuries didn't occur simultaneously, they did occur one after the other. Each doctor kept Bear on a regiment of steroids for an extended period of time. Bear, already a large man, ballooned up to over 400 pounds. So, at the time that we received the news that Bear had Type II diabetes and had Chronic Kidney Disease, he was also morbidly obese. It was going to be along hard road.

Chronic Kidney Disease is a degenerative disease. In extremely rare cases, the kidney regains function. But, for the most part, once they start to fail, it is only a matter of time before the go completely. At that point, the patient must go through dialysis treatments multiple times a week. We received counseling from dialysis nutritionists. The diet that they encouraged my husband to eat was atrocious. Diet soda, white bread, and a host of other processed foods were not only allowed, but encouraged! I was going to use all my education and research to bear on the fight we had before us.

The first thing I did was to eliminate processed foods. If I couldn't pronounce every ingredient in my food, it didn't go in my pantry. Gluten was eliminated. My studies showed me that it is a tremendous inflammatory. Guess how he acquired gout? Sugar as we know it was gone. Instead, we went with coconut sugar, honey, molasses, and other natural sweeteners. On the rare occasions when I made pancakes for him, we used pure maple syrup. I could hear the head of his endocrinologist (the doctor treating him for diabetes) explode as I watched my husband enjoy this wonderful treat.

We went to organic locally-grown fruits and vegetables. My belief is that not only are they higher in nutrients than their GMO counterparts, but they are safer to eat due to the lack of residual pesticides and their genetic integrity. When we ate meats, they would be from grass feed cows, and free-range pigs and chickens. These meats provide proteins that are devoid of the hormones and antibiotics that are forced into non-free-range meats.

Our dairy came straight from the farmer. We ate free-range eggs, and lots of them! I could feel his doctors cringe as we told them he was eating at least two eggs a day with nitrate-free bacon. We drank raw milk, complete with all the fat that those wonderful cows give us. We ate raw cheese. The nutritionists and doctors were going to have coronaries of their own when they heard the direction we were taking.

Our first dreaded meeting with a nutritionist was made at the dialysis center. She ran through a list of FDA mandated dietary guidelines and suggestions. As she spoke, I politely replied, "No. We will not be doing that." She became more and more infuriated and frustrated with me until she finally snorted, "Well, I guess we'll see when that lab work gets in!" Yes we would. We had one month before the next lab report. We were going to make the most of the time before us.

During that month, we followed the prescribed plan. Eat real food. That was what this was going to be all about. We ate organic locally-grown fruits and vegetables, organic free-range meats, natural sugars, whole grains, and supplements. One of the supplements added was Tumeric, a powerful anti-inflammatory. Cinnamon, a wonderful tool in naturally lowering blood sugar, was, also, added. Probiotics and digestive enzymes were additionally added. And, when we washed down our meals, it was with cool, clear water. Sodas were strictly forbidden. By doing this, we were able to lower his prescription drug intake from 12 to three.

His lab work was drawn and the day to meet with our doctor and nutritionist was at hand. The news was remarkable. His A1C had gone from 8.7 to 6.3. It was now just above the normal range of 6.0. The argument of not being able to eat something wholesome and sweet was now mute. His cholesterol had gone from a total of 202 to 155. Bacon, eggs, and whole dairy products are not the villain they have been made out to be. It was with no small amount of joy that I received the nutritionist's comment, "Well, I guess I can't tell *you* anything." That's right! I'll be eating real food!

Interspersed with whole, real food, I would give my husband some smoothies to enhance his nutrition. Foods that he was not fond of eating could be consumed through a smoothie. As the saying goes, "A spoonful of sugar helps the medicine go down." So, with his kale-spinach-goji berry-cacao-nib-carrot-chia-flaxseed-molasses-apple-banana-broccoli-blueberry smoothie, I would add some coconut sugar. This book will not allow me to detail the density of the nutrition in this smoothie, but trust me when I tell you this will make you healthy as a horse!

Now, I love my husband with all my heart. But, I have to be honest. He has always had a voracious appetite. He loves to say that after eating a rib-eye, the thing he likes most for dessert is another rib-eye. He was so concerned about his appetite that he actually thought there was something medically wrong. A doctor was going to prescribe him a $200 per month drug to trick his brain into thinking he was full. Fortunately, my husband never took the prescription. However, as my husband began to change his eating habits, something quite interesting began to happen. He started feeling full . . . . and while eating less food!

You see, what was happening was that my husband was eating more nutrient-dense foods. As that started to take hold in his body, his brain started to realize that the body was getting what it needed. As the body was getting what it needed, the brains told the body it was O.K. to stop eating. When we eat junk food, or food that has no real nutritional value, we continue to eat until we bust. And, even then, we want to eat just a short time later. Why? Because we have not ingested the nutrients the body needs to function properly. As a result, my husband started to drop weight. And he wasn't really trying very hard at all.

Here we are one year later. Bear's cholesterol is still in the 150's, his A1C stays in the low 5's, and he has dropped over 100 pounds. He is still on dialysis. But his doctor's say that he is the healthiest kidney patient around. He is working hard to get on a kidney list. In order to do so, he must be a certain weight. He is almost there. We will continue to work hard to get there, get a transplant, and get on with our lives.

Our success in managing my husband's disease has been the catalyst for me to get the message of health through whole foods out to the community. I continue to coach and counsel others in their wellness journeys. Their maladies may be different. But, the treatment is essentially the same. Eat whole foods in their original state. Eat your medicine. Eat yourself to life!

Health is a choice. Every time you consume something, whether it is food or drink, you make a choice. We can choose to nourish our bodies with fuel that will make us strong and feel great. Or, we can ingest something that will fill our stomachs, but do nothing to help our body function at peak levels. We waited until it was almost too late before we did something to change our lives. We don't ever want to see anyone live through the events that we lived, and currently live, through. And, you don't have to. Learn from our trials and live well.

About Brandie Schwartz

Brandie Schwartz CHHC, AADP, RNWCON, is from Odessa, Texas. Most of her life has been dedicated to health and caring for others. She started volunteering at Medical Center Hospital in Odessa in 1990. This led to her pursuit of a nursing career. She graduated from Odessa College with her Registered Nursing license in 1994. In 1996, Brandie graduated from University of Texas, Permian Basin with her Bachelor's Degree in Nursing. For the next 16 years, nursing was her career. She moved to California to marry her husband, Bear, in 2002. In 2008, they moved to Springfield, Missouri.

*She is a graduate of The Institute for Integrative Nutrition where she became a Certified Holistic Health Coach. Brandie owns and operates **Eat Your Medicine** (www.http://eatyourmedicine.info). As a health coach, she serves as a mentor to help people make healthy life style choices and achieve personal wellness goals. Whether the desired outcome is weight loss, boosted energy levels, improved digestion, or the treatment of a chronic condition, Brandie focuses on the individual needs of each client and work within the realities of their day-to-day challenges. By helping clients make manageable behavioral changes that can be maintained over time, she empowers people to take responsibility for their own health and achieve optimal wellness.*

*In addition to running **Eat Your Medicine** and taking care of her husband, Brandie is the proud mother of two sons, Caleb and Garret.*

In the sick room, ten cents' worth of human understanding equals ten dollars' worth of medical science. ~Martin H. Fischer

Next up, learn what your fertility doctor WON'T tell you about how to conceive naturally without spending thousands on artificial fertilization methods. There is a way! Read Mare Pulido's account of how natural medicine made her pregnancy dream come true!

Meet a woman who was told she could not get pregnant without help from artificial insemination or in vitro fertilization methods. Lucky for her, natural medicine enabled her to conceive a child without 'outside help' and she is now the grateful mother of a beautiful daughter.

From Infertile to A Beautiful Baby Girl: How I Conceived Naturally When My Doctors Told Me I Couldn't

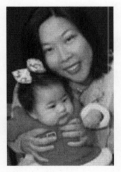

by Mare Pulido, http://holisticmamas.com

When I first started out on the path of natural healing and educating myself on modalities like herbs and aromatherapy, I had no idea of the kind of journey it would take me on!

These holistic health alternatives have helped me better service my wellness spa customers, aided me in conceiving a child and fulfilling my lifelong dream of becoming a Mom, and supported me in my quest to keep my daughter healthy without resorting to potentially harmful conventional means. I hope my story will resonate with you and your own journey towards natural health!

I first got interested in natural medicine and herbal remedies while owning a wellness spa. One of the highlights of my day was dreaming up new services that would both relax my clients as well as provide therapeutic benefits for them. I would salivate over the chance to attend trade shows and vendor-offered courses to learn more about seaweed wraps, herbal teas, essential oils-based skin and body care, and more. I couldn't get enough of it.

During my spa-owning years, I took full advantage of the tax write-off to fill out my education in alternative health, earning a certification in Aromatherapy and a Master Herbalist diploma from what is now the American College of Healthcare Sciences.

I saw firsthand how the treatments I had designed helped my clients. Some of my favorites included the "Deep Forest Detox," a body wrap service that used oils of Pine, Cypress, Juniper, Cedarwood, and Lemon to help the body rid itself of toxins, and the "Spice and Ice" facial, which used the natural rubefacient properties of Paprika to give skin a luminous glow.

Instead of hurrying clients out after a massage, I had my staff gently wake them up with a little "Peppermint Head Trip" (a quick scalp massage using a drop of Peppermint essential oil), which served the dual purpose of rejuvenating them AND getting them out of the room quickly so the next client could begin.

I felt incredibly fulfilled whenever a client would tell me of some physical ailment and I could devise a remedy for it. One day, "Jane" complained of being stuffed up before her pedicure, and I prepared a Eucalyptus steam inhalation for her that she could enjoy while getting her toes polished. Afterwards, she said her sinuses had cleared and she felt refreshed.

When "Kathy" complained of a cold, I hand-blended her a tea containing Sage, Chamomile, and Thyme, three very good herbs for producing sweat (which comes in handy during a cold). Later, she sent me a note letting me know how much it had helped her, and asking where she could buy that blend in the supermarket.

"Sheila" often had gas and constipation, so I prepared a tea containing Licorice root, Cinnamon, Ginger, Peppermint, and Fennel, a potent combination for stimulating peristalsis—a fancy word for "getting things moving" in the pipes. The best part was, it tasted delicious, too.

It seemed that I had discovered my life's passion as a result of operating the spa. But in the midst of all this spa-owning bliss, my husband and I began to yearn for a child. We tried off and on to conceive for years, without any success. Finally, after five frustrating years of trying, we went to see a well-known and highly recommended fertility doctor, who shall remain nameless in this account.

I'll never forget that awful, defeating, and demoralizing day. She told me that I had less than 2% chance of conceiving on my own, and after viewing them on ultrasound, let me know that my ovaries were—and I quote—"sad-looking." I felt angry and patronized. I wanted to ask her, "Is that a clinical term that you learned in medical school?"

Because of our low probability of conceiving, she suggested that we try artificial insemination, and if that did not work, in vitro fertilization

(IVF). But in order to go that route, I would have to first get an HSG (a hysterosalpingogram), a process during which they would inject dye into my uterus to scan for fibroids or blockages. And in order to have an HSG, I would have to take several days of antibiotics to minimize the risk of infection.

And finally, because I did not have insurance coverage for fertility (the insurance choices for small business owners are not exactly robust in this country), I would have to self-fund the procedure, which for the HSG alone was approximately $2,000. I cried the entire way home, and the following day, left for Las Vegas on business, and cried the entire way there. It was September 2008, and I felt like I had hit an emotional rock bottom.

I agonized over whether to undergo that procedure. The strange thing was, the money is not what bothered me—I knew I could eventually scrape together the funds for it. No, it was the thought of taking antibiotics that had created such an internal conflict within me. I really didn't want to subject my body to that, and I resisted the thought with every cell I had. Luckily, I had (and have) an extremely loving husband, who respected me and told me he would support whatever decision I made. We decided to put the procedure on hold, and started to consider adoption.

After selecting our adoption agency and going through the initial steps and educational seminar, the only thing left to do was fill out the giant binder of adoption paperwork to begin the process. I don't know what prevented my husband and I from filling it out, but the thing just sat on our coffee table for months, gathering layer upon layer of dust. Perhaps we really were not that motivated to adopt a child after all. Regardless, around May of 2009, I had an epiphany: I believed sincerely in alternative and natural medicine—it was the foundation of my healing philosophy at my wellness spa. Why, then, had I not thought about applying it to fertility and my inability to conceive?

In June of 2009, I went to see Dr. Connie Hernandez, a naturopathic doctor who specialized in women's medicine. She immediately put me at ease, and told me that we would first take a full blood panel to find out if I had sufficient hormone levels or any thyroid deficiencies (all I remember is an alphabet soup of acronyms like TSH and FSH). The blood panel showed that all of my levels were normal—in fact, they were "optimal"—but that my Vitamin D level was "out-of-sight low." Dr. Hernandez explained to me that without sufficient Vitamin D, I would not be able to conceive, let alone carry a pregnancy to term. Therefore, we began a regimen of 5,000 IUs of Vitamin D per day.

Also, she suggested that I strengthen the connection between my brain and my ovaries. To do that, she gave me Maca root powder and Vitex extract. Maca root powder is by far the most disgusting substance I have ever had—I would rather lick the bottom of someone's sweaty feet than take it again, but I simply had to do it. I would roll it together with honey, carob powder, and shredded coconut to try to make SOMETHING edible out of it, but no matter what I tried, it still tasted terrible.

We also decided to strengthen my liver, so I used castor oil hot packs and a liver supporting medicine (SLF Forte was the name of it, as I recall) to help with that endeavor.

Dr. Hernandez also suggested alternating sitz baths of hot and cold water. My husband would fill up two tubs—one of hot water and one cold. I would first sit with my butt in the hot water, and my feet in the cold. After 3 minutes of that, I would then switch, putting my butt in the cold water and my feet in the hot water for 30 seconds (seriously, it was all I could stand anyway). Finally, we also decided to use flower essences to help align my emotional and spiritual energies with this endeavor. Dr. Hernandez hand-mixed it herself and gave me an affirmation to use daily: "I now become a vessel for the highest good of the Universe."

Hallelujah! By late October 2009, I was pregnant! I spent the next nine months in a state of extreme joy. My pregnancy was about as smooth as a pregnancy could be—I felt great, slept well, ate well, and generally wished I could go around pregnant all the time.

All was well in my life, except the economy. By 2010, my spa was operating at one-third of the revenue level we enjoyed in 2006, and I fell further and further behind in meeting my financial obligations. Finally, my landlord sent me a termination of tenancy letter that asked me to move out by the end of June 2010.

But even the loss of my business was unable to dampen my happiness. On August 2, 2010, I gave birth to my miracle daughter, Aria. She was (and is) the culmination of my life, my dreams-made-flesh, and natural medicine had helped me to get there. I became a passionate proponent of holistic medicine, telling my story to anyone who would listen. Eventually, I decided to just start blogging about it, as well as about any holistic and natural remedies that I used to take care of my daughter. I never thought I would join the legions of mommy bloggers in the world, but here I am, and loving it.

My daughter's early months were quite rough for me. We had trouble getting breastfeeding going because she had a "tongue tie," so at 9 days old, she endured the surgical procedure to release it. After that, she refused to breastfeed and would arch her back (away from the breast) and cry at the top of her lungs whenever I would try to nurse her. She also would exhibit this behavior late at night, arching her back and crying as if in extreme pain for hours on end.

My husband and I were at the end of our proverbial ropes: sleep-deprived, exhausted, helpless, and hopeless. When we took her to her pediatrician at 4 weeks old, we were told that she had reflux, a condition that allowed some of her stomach acids to come back into her esophagus or mouth, causing extreme pain. For this, the doctor prescribed a baby antacid.

I was told to administer it to her until she was 4 to 6 months old, and as you might expect, the "natural mama" in me rebelled. I was NOT going to give my child a medicine that would effectively suppress acid production, as I reasoned that she needed those acids for good digestion. But I was also in a bind, because my training as a Master Herbalist taught me that we cannot give herbs to children under two because their livers lack the enzymes to properly process them. Nor could I give her any essential oils for basically the same reason.

I began to research natural remedies online with a passion, completely ignoring the wisdom to "sleep when the baby sleeps." I was determined to get my baby off of the antacid as soon as possible.

That's when I came across Homeopathy, the healing discipline of using "like to heal like." The idea behind homeopathy is that large doses of a substance can cause symptoms in a healthy person, but small—I should say, micro-doses—of that same substance can heal those same symptoms in a sick person. No one really knows why this works, not even homeopaths (although the theories abound), but it often does.

I bought a homeopathy handbook and began learning about remedies. I learned that each remedy had its own symptom picture, and to use homeopathy properly, you matched up the symptoms with the remedy that addressed the most symptoms. That was how I came across *Dioscorea villosa*, the remedy that seemed to match the most of my daughter's reflux symptoms (arching of the back, worse lying down, worse at night, and so on and so forth). However, I didn't have any *Dioscorea* on hand, and neither did the nearby pharmacy. I had to send away for it, but in the meantime, I used the next best thing I had in hand: *Nux Vomica*.

Suffice it to say that it took a week for the *Discorea* remedy to get to me, but by then, my daughter was already completely asymptomatic of reflux, and already entirely off of "Baby Zantac." She was 5 weeks old, and interestingly enough, that was also the week that we had our first successful breastfeeding session. It turned out that the pain of lying sideways prevented her from nursing, and when I had solved the pain, we were able to begin a long and mutually satisfying breastfeeding relationship.

If I had to share one piece of wisdom with moms who want to use natural medicine to help care for their families, I would tell them to do their own research and develop their own support networks. When it comes to your child's health, it is important to become as highly educated as possible about all of the choices out there.

If you want to use alternative medicine to care for your child, then you will need to seek out as many credible resources as possible—texts, online informational web sites, medical and herbal research, professional practitioners like homeopaths, naturopaths, osteopaths, etc., and other like-minded moms. Doing copious amounts of research and listening to my fellow "natural moms" have been the cornerstones of my success in keeping my little Aria happy and healthy.

Following my heart's desire to learn more about natural health and wellness has helped me make my dreams come true. Without embarking on this path, I might not have been able to become a mother or take care of my daughter successfully with alternative, non-harmful means. I hope you have been inspired to explore natural medicine and the many ways it can help create blessings for you and your family.

About Mare Pulido, M.H.

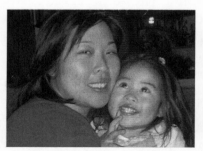

Mare is a Master Herbalist and Certified Aromatherapist who enjoys writing about natural health and using holistic home remedies to create therapeutic benefits for her husband, Angelo, and daughter, Aria. By day, she leads digital marketing and online strategy for a technology company, and by night she shares her experiences in natural parenting via the Holistic Mamas blog.

The art of medicine consists in amusing the patient while nature cures the disease.

~Voltaire

Coming along next is a woman who shares her love for Red Raspberry Leaf Tea. This simple herb is a woman's best friend. It's wonderful benefits during and after childbirth and for the common aches and discomforts of PMS is truly incredible. Learn how to make your own simple tea and love being a woman.

Red Raspberry Tea:
A Woman's Best Friend

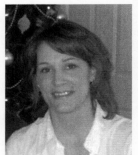

by Paula J. Miller, http://www.WholeIntentions.com

Pain has been around since the beginning of time.

Pain from PMS, cramping during menstruation, childbirth, and all those wonderful things, come with being female. I came to the conclusion early in 'womanhood' that this was simply a fact of life. Women would endure pain.

Mankind and conventional medicine has come up with all sorts of ways to deal with this aspect of a woman's life: Tylenol, Aleve, birth control, epidurals, etc. As a menstruating teenager I embraced these methods with little thought. I assumed that doctors knew best, painkillers were something I could enjoy (my poor, poor ancestors!), and there really wasn't much more to consider.

I'm not a wimp, but I wouldn't say I have high pain tolerance either. I gladly took pain killers during my first several deliveries. And while I had those tiny toes to distract me, the after pains did a good job of bringing me out of my baby-kissed delirium and back to the present—and a bottle of pain relief pills.

But life has a way of changing things.

Through severe morning sickness during each pregnancy, a sudden and unexplained stillbirth, my husband's mysterious health symptoms which increased with each passing year, and other seemingly random health concerns, the light started to dawn.

We'd turned to a myriad of doctors, but were fed up with the answers they gave us. Finally, we began doing our own digging. Using well-researched books, the internet, homeopathic doctors, forums . . . we read and pondered healthcare and medicine for several years. In the end, we came up with the startling realization that conventional medicine didn't have all the answers.

By the time I was 8 months along with our fifth baby, I'd learned enough about the dangers of pain meds given during childbirth that I was determined to go through future labors and delivery without them. Of course, I didn't dwell too long on what that would actually entail. I just knew what my plan was—and I was sticking to it!

When an herbalist friend told me about red raspberry tea, a safe and natural drink that was beneficial in making labor easier and shorter, I waddled across the floor and practically tackled her!

Let's just say she got me on the 'easier' and 'shorter' part.

I bought the tea, and according to her recommendations, drank however much I wanted. I started out well, but in all honestly it was a bit hard to believe a tea could make that much difference. I decided to drink it for health's sake, and not expect too much.

My drug-free labor produced a beautiful baby boy, along with the startling realization that either I was getting senile or the pain of childbirth wasn't nearly as bad as I thought it would be. I mean, it wasn't a walk in the park—but I noticed a definite difference compared to my other deliveries.

Mothering four little boys soon took over my life however, and I didn't give the tea much more thought.

My husband's newly discovered food allergies took up a large majority of my time and research, but we were slowly and surely headed down the 'healthy living' road.

Then, surprise! Two years later we found ourselves expecting again. I remembered the red raspberry leaf tea my friend had recommended and started reading. If the little I drank during my previous pregnancy could make me raise my eyebrows in pleasant surprise, what could an entire pregnancy's worth do?

I started drinking it cold, like iced tea, and by my second trimester I was drinking it in earnest. I couldn't get enough! I could easily down a quart a day—I craved it. And while I guzzled, I read every blog, article, and forum I could find. I was amazed and encouraged by the health benefits and testimonies women were sharing.

I was ready to embrace natural medicine.

How did it affect my delivery?

My Braxton Hicks, which in previous pregnancies started around 5 months, didn't begin until 37 weeks.

Then about 1:00 a.m., two days after my due date, I noticed they were coming about ten minutes apart. They were light, which was typical, but they were also consistent—which wasn't typical.

Finally, I woke my husband at 2:30 a.m. and we decided to head to the hospital. The drive was 45 min. but I'd read him so many stories about how the tea encourages quick labor that we made it in just under 27 min.

When we checked in at 3:45 a.m. I was only 1 cm dilated. Within an hour I'd progressed to 4 cm, and after another hour I was at 5 cm. I was surprised at how quickly I was progressing since my contractions were barely any worse than the ones that woke me that morning. In fact, I was disappointed they were so light—I wanted to get the show on the road!

Finally they became strong enough that I asked to sit in the bathtub.

I got into the bathtub at 6:00 a.m. but the warm water didn't seem to help. I wasn't in the bathtub very long when I told my husband I wanted to get out. As soon as I stood up, I felt the urge to push.

By time I'd tottered back to the bed I was 9 ½ cm. Three pushes later our daughter was born on the end of the bed at 6:20 a.m. When the doctor ran into the room, we were already oohing and ahhing over her.

What surprised me the most, was that after nearly 5 hours of labor, my contractions were still 'do-able'—and the last 10 minutes went amazingly fast.

I won't lie and say the tea made the after pains non-existent, but I certainly noticed a difference. By the third day the pains were pretty much gone and my husband couldn't stop commenting on how much better I looked and how much more energy I had. I'd never felt so good after delivery!

Red Raspberry Leaf Tea and PMS

For as long as I could remember I'd have heavy periods that lasted nearly two weeks from beginning to end. My cramping made me miserable, and my mood swings didn't help anyone!

In the research I'd done during my pregnancy, I found that this tea was beneficial for more than just labor and delivery. The many references to PMS, cramping, and its ability to reduce a heavy flow made me continue drinking it for the 14 months I breastfed.

When my periods started coming back again, I could hardly believe it. They were 'text book' periods: seven days from start to finish, a much, much lighter flow, and nearly a perfect 28 day cycle. In fact, they were so different than my previous periods I began to worry that something was wrong!

It's been three years since we had our daughter, and I've become convinced (as has my husband!) that the red raspberry leaf tea is an essential part of nurturing your female reproductive organs and hormones.

The Benefits of Red Raspberry Leaf Tea

It's often amazing to me how herbs like this one could be created and used for thousands of years and then suddenly they're questioned, discouraged, and eventually forgotten for more 'modern' solutions. I used to feel pity for my medicine-less ancestors, but now I realize they had the use of the best medicines of all!

It still astounds me at the treasure trove inside simple and delicious red raspberry leaf tea. It:

- increases fertility in both men and women
- eases morning sickness
- strengthens and tones the entire female reproductive system
- acts as an amazing uterine toner due to the presence of an alkaloid called fragrine. Fragrine allows the uterus to contract more powerfully and effectively during labor. The muscles don't consume all their oxygen which results in less contractions, less straining, and less effort from the muscles - and therefore less cramping sensations. Basically it allows the uterus to work more efficiently.
- reduces incidences of artificial rupturing of membranes, forceps delivery, or cesarean births
- aids in toning the uterus after birth as it returns back to its usual size
- decreases profuse menstrual flow
- helps relieve cramping during menstrual cycles

Not only are the leaves a good uterine tonic, it's also high in both zinc and manganese. Zinc is known for shortening labor, strengthening connective tissue, preventing nipple cracks, bonding, avoiding post partum depression and preventing inconsolable crying in babies. Manganese is a mineral that helps form bones and cartilage.

Red raspberry leaves also contain an easily assimilated form of calcium which is necessary in controlling nerve response to pain during childbirth as well as aiding bone development in the baby. The high vitamin and mineral content helps to replace those that are lost via blood during delivery.

Midwives often say drinking red raspberry tea is "watering the soil"—growing a really healthy placenta to nourish the baby. They encourage women to start drinking 1-2 cups a day during their second trimester and then the sky's the limit! A quart a day is comparable to a day's worth of leafy greens.

How Do You Make Red Raspberry Leaf Tea?

Here's a simple recipe I follow:

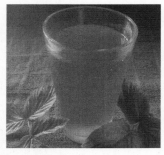

    8 parts red raspberry leaves
    3 parts alfalfa
    3 parts peppermint (if you're nursing, replace this with fenugreek as peppermint can decrease your milk supply)
    2 parts nettles

Alfalfa, peppermint, and nettles each add their own benefits. Mixed with red raspberry tea, it makes a safe but powerful herbal remedy for a myriad of issues.

Directions:

1. Combine herbs and store in an air tight jar or container.
2. To make a single serving of hot tea, pour a cup of boiling water over 1-2 teaspoons of the tea mix. Let it steep for about 5 min. Remove the leaves or strain the tea and sweeten it with stevia or another natural sweetener.
3. To make a large batch of cold tea (my favorite), pour about 4 cups of boiling water over ½ c. of the loose leaves and let it steep for about 4 hours.
4. Strain the leaves and pour the condensed tea liquid into a gallon container.
5. Sweeten with stevia or another natural sweetener and fill the gallon the rest of the way with water. Place it in the refrigerator until cold. This tastes great on a hot day!

No Regrets

I don't regret the way in which I've learned about natural remedies. Sixteen years ago as a carefree and clueless newlywed, someone could have handed me a book with every herb and remedy there was and I wouldn't have known the value I held.

Until we each face our own health issues, or someone we loves suffers from eczema, allergies, insomnia, ADHD, etc. and we come to the place that we realize we don't like the answers we've been handed, most of the talk about natural medicine goes in one ear and out the other. I've been there too!

If life didn't taken the turns it does, we would all be indifferent to learning how to take care of our bodies and those of our loved ones. We wouldn't have the joy of discovering age-old answers that have been tucked away for thousands of years. And our families won't reap the benefits of safe and natural remedies.

Can you imagine? Had men and women not passed down their secrets and recipes throughout the generations, we'd be sitting here, dependent on modern medicine, chemical drugs, and unnecessary procedures—and not knowing any different.

You can take care of yourself and your family. You can research carefully and learn new subjects that you might have never considered before. It doesn't matter how old you are, how new you are to the idea of natural health, or how many PhD's you have behind your name. The joy and wonder of using God's gifts of nature never loses its thrill.

The answers to a wonderful birthing experience, less post-partum pain, easier PMS symptoms, and a lighter and shorter flow are packed into an unsuspecting green leaf we usually ignore when reaching for plump, red berries. The joys of being a woman are within your reach, and in a tall glass of tea.

About Paula Miller

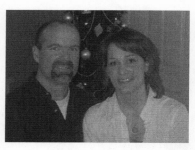
Paula is the wife of 16 years to her beloved husband as well as a homeschooling mother to their five children. Several years of family health problems centered around a stillbirth, Lyme's Disease, and food allergies created a passion to learn about nourishing foods, Candida, fitness, and healthy alternatives to modern medicine.

She's turned her passion and research into a way to help others learn about the benefits of natural living. She chats about whole food, whole living, and whole faith at www.WholeIntentions.com. When she can, she likes to mix in homesteading, gardening, and healthy doses of coconut oil.

Life begins where your comfort zone ends.
~Neale Donald Walsch

Next up, Cara Nitz will show you how to have the birthing story you always envisioned! She would like to share her drug-free home birth with you, helping you understand how a natural birth can do more than just give you a beautiful story. So, turn the page and read more . . .

Proud, Strong, and Confident:
Why I Decided To Go With a Natural Birth

by *Cara Nitz,* http://yourworldnatural.blogspot.com

Here is my story. The story of a woman who was just an average "Jane." I ate the standard American diet, exercised, but had many health problems. Follow my journey through healing, hope, one nightmare of a birth story, two beautiful home birth stories, and what I learned along the way.

I grew up knowing little about health and natural living. I learned a little bit as I went through adolescence and tried to stay in shape and good health through college. However, my health still suffered from my diet and lifestyle choices, which were the same as the average American.

By the time I was married, I had been on birth control as a way to get my monthly cycle to return after a full year of not getting it. I had been on depression medication. I had been to see doctor after doctor about recurring stomach pains, migraines, and joint pain. No one seemed to know what to do other than to prescribe more medication.

After my husband and I struggled for a little over a year to get pregnant, we finally found ourselves having our first child—a boy. While I was starting to learn a little bit about natural, healthy living, I still had a lot to learn.

The pregnancy and birth of my son was far from what I had imagined it to be. My pregnancy was full of fainting spells, severe nausea, migraine headaches, and more. My labor was nightmarish and ended with an epidural, which was the last thing I had wanted.

My labor started as my water broke while I was in the bathtub. After we arrived at the hospital about an hour later, the contractions were getting stronger. They were all in my back, and they got to be very intense within a couple hours. While I tried walking, hot showers, heat packs, nothing seemed to help. The pain was so intense that I vomited several times. After enduring these contractions for almost 20 hours, I was so physically exhausted and the pain was so intense I ended up getting a dose of pain medicine which did nothing and then followed that with an epidural. Four hours later, I had my beautiful baby boy in my arms, and my heart overflowed with love and joy! Fast forward a couple weeks, and despite the fact that I started nursing him as soon as possible, I was unable to provide my son with enough milk and ended up supplementing with formula.

I was and still am disappointed that I had to resort to having an epidural, which I believe is dangerous to my health and my baby's health. I also am disappointed with the fact that I had to supplement my nursing with formula, which I believe may be caused in part by the epidural and lack of nutrients and/or protein in my diet.

I was determined to make a change in my life and take control of my health and the health of my future children.

In the 2 ½ years between my first and second child, I switched out all my conventional, toxic cleaners and personal care products for safer, green, organic versions. I started eating cleaner, organic food. I took supplements and vitamins to give my body what it needed to thrive.

When we started trying to get pregnant with our second child, we got pregnant much faster and easier. And my daughter's birth was the complete opposite of my son's birth. When I found out I was pregnant, I was determined to have a different birth story than last time. I wanted to labor in the comfortable and natural surroundings of my own home. I also wanted a midwife that would support what I believed about birth—that it is a natural process and not one that needs to be medicated and treated as an illness or medical problem.

I found a fabulous homebirth midwife and started seeing her while I was in my first trimester. Throughout the pregnancy, she cared for me as a daughter. She recommended natural solutions to my nausea and gave me ideas for how to have a healthy, safe pregnancy. The result was a much smoother, healthier pregnancy with no migraines, no fainting and less nausea. My labor was a new and different experience that I found myself looking back on with pride, fond memories, and peace.

A week after my due date, my midwife suggested sitting on my birthing ball, crawling on all fours, and a few other natural ways of getting labor started. I used all her suggestions, and my labor started in the middle of the night with contractions about 3-4 minutes apart. I called my midwife, and she drove over immediately.

After the midwives arrived, I spent the next 7 hours or so sitting on my birthing ball swaying my hips side to side, breathing through each contraction. This was definitely not like my last child's birth! This time, I was in the comfort of my own home, in my pajamas, reading a book between contractions, watching the sunrise, listening to my CD of birds and nature sounds, chatting with my son when he woke up, and feeling overall strong, peaceful, and comfortable in my surroundings. My midwives went to sleep to give me as much space as I worked with my body through labor. I moved in and out of different rooms, had my morning protein shake, didn't have to worry about new nurses always coming and going, monitors and IV's stuck on and in me. I felt so at ease, even though it was still painful.

After being in labor for a little over seven hours, my midwife checked me for the first time, and I was at 7 cm. Contractions were getting worse and worse, and she said that if I wanted them to break my water, they would. I waited awhile longer, and then they broke my water. I sat on the birthing stool to get a feel for if that was how I wanted to start pushing, but it was uncomfortable to me. So, I moved back into the shower, and through all the pain, ended up on the floor of the shower ready to push.

I moved out back to the birthing stool—not comfortable, and onto my side on my bed (which they had covered very well with plastic sheets and pads). I pushed a little while like that, but then ended up pushing my little daughter out on my bed. It turned out she had her arm up with her head, which made it a lot harder to push her out. My midwives were great with warm compresses and such to help me from not tearing, and I ended up with only a little tiny tear, most likely because of the extra hand and arm that she stuck out.

I had done it!!! I gave birth in the most natural setting I can think of—my own home with no drugs or other interventions with my wonderful encouraging midwives. They helped me so much without being pushy or in the way. They offered so many words of strength and love. I feel blessed to have had them at my daughter's birth!

An hour or two after the birth, the midwives prepared an herbal bath for me to go in with my baby. It helped with healing me and my battle wounds, and it helps with the baby's cord to dry up faster and heal well. It was a special, relaxing time for my daughter and I.

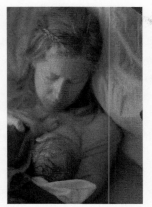

My midwives were also extremely supportive and helpful in starting breastfeeding. They gave me lots of herbal teas to help boost my milk supply and really helped her to latch on the right way soon after she was born. I had no problems with breastfeeding this time, and I loved being able to feed my baby all on my own, giving her all the nourishment that she needed!

Things went just as well, if not better, with my third child's birth.

After being three weeks overdue, my labor finally started at about 4 am. I had been having contractions for weeks, but the contractions that woke me up at 4 am were much sharper and concentrated more in my lower back. I knew these were different. I started timing them at about 10 minutes apart, so I called my midwife. After getting some excited encouragement from my midwife, I hopped in the shower, and when I got out, my contractions had jumped to about 3 minutes apart! So, I called my midwife again to give her an update and she scurried over.

I jumped back in the shower, because standing with the water hitting my back, swaying and keeping my body relaxed made most of the pain go away. This was a night and day difference from my first pregnancy in the hospital.

After getting out of the shower and saying hello to my midwife, I sat on my stability ball for a couple hours, while my two other children woke up and had breakfast. They got just as excited as I was seeing the midwife and knowing that the baby was coming soon! It was very comforting for me to spend time with my children and family while I labored. We had fun listening to the nature sounds CD that I also listened to through my last home birth with my other daughter.

I fueled my body a bit with some peanut butter toast and plenty of fluids, which tasted great! Then, I headed back to the shower, since the contractions were getting worse. My husband stayed in the bathroom with me and rubbed my back through each contraction, which helped a bit too. After awhile, I decided I wanted to be checked by the midwife, so she checked heartbeat and dilation. I was so happy to be 8 cm dilated and to hear that the baby was doing fantastic. However, the baby's head was still pretty high, so I decided to try laying in the child's pose to get the baby to come down. Through each contraction, I kept coaching myself to relax—from my fingertips to my toes—and I think that really helped to get through them without going insane.

After a while longer, I got checked again and was 10 cm and ready to push. I tried several different positions, including squatting on the birth stool, standing, lying on my side. After 30 minutes, we decided something was holding the baby up, so I lay on my back on my bed, got my knees way up and pushed as hard as I possibly could for 2 straight minutes to get her out. It was fast, furious, and outrageously painful, but it worked. Out she came and then we saw the reason for the hold up. My little stinker had her arm up and around her head, which made the pushing process much harder.

I immediately received my daughter to hold on my chest, and I was just shocked, once again, to see my little miracle for the first time! She was beautiful and perfect and had a great cry right from the get-go!

As I gazed at my beautiful daughter, I felt intense pain from the powerful pushing phase, which must have caused many abrasions "down there." It felt like a million stabbing knives and my whole body couldn't stop shaking. After about a half hour or so, (plus warm compresses, gentle music playing to calm me down, lots of deep breaths) the pain started to lessen a bit, and I was able to start nursing my baby. She latched on pretty quickly, which was another relief.

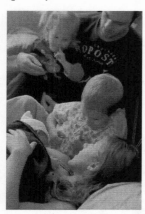
After nursing for awhile, my children came in to meet their new little sister, my midwife did the newborn exam, and then my baby and I enjoyed a nice herbal bath to soothe and heal us both.

I know it made a huge difference in my last two births that I made my own health a priority and trusted in natural remedies to alleviate any struggles through pregnancy and childbirth. Where most doctors would prescribe medication, my midwife offered natural plant and herbal remedies. With my last daughter's birth, when she wasn't coming out with normal pushing and seemed to be stuck, most doctors probably would have told me I couldn't give birth naturally and had to have a C-section. Instead, I had faith that my body was meant to do this, and I pushed her out, despite her arm being wrapped around her head. Instead of telling me that breastfeeding may not work and offering formula to feed my baby, my midwife supported and believed in my body's ability, recommending nettle, alfalfa and raspberry leaf teas for healthy breastfeeding and healing after my births.

Thanks to natural remedies, my last two births were wonderful experiences that left me feeling proud, strong, and even more confident in natural medicine and my ability to know what my body needed. Best of all, I have been blessed with three beautiful, healthy children who fill my home and life with joy!

As my for my own health, I haven't been on depression medication since my first child's birth, and all my stomach issues and pain are completely gone. I still have the occasional joint pain, but it is much less painful and much rarer. And I am happy to say that I am migraine free! It is amazing what a difference it makes when you use natural remedies and supply your body with what it needs to thrive!

I hope I have sparked something inside of you. I hope to have given you clarity on why it is so important to take control of your health, be your own advocate and fight for what you know is best for you and your family. Fill your lives with people who support you in providing your family with natural alternatives. The more you nourish yourself with things that come from nature and not those developed in a lab, the more you will thrive. As you have seen from my story, it is possible to come from a place of suffering and pain to a place of growth and joy through natural alternatives.

About Cara Nitz

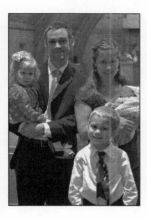

Cara Nitz is a mother of three, wife, fitness instructor, personal trainer health coach and blogger. She has a degree in Elementary Education with an emphasis on Physical Education. Since her first child was born, she has fed her passion for healthy living by learning even more about nutrition, fitness, natural products, and ways to keep our homes and families safe and healthy. She feels it is a real blessing in her life to share what she knows with others. It gives her the greatest joy to impact other people's lives in a positive and wonderful way!

A mother always has to think twice,
once for herself and once for her child.

–Sophia Loren

You won't want to miss the next chapter, where Kristy Howard outlines baby steps for natural mothering! Have you ever felt skeptical about herbs or natural living? You'll read about a mama who started out her motherhood career as an indifferent skeptic, and ended up an aspiring herbalist! Not surprisingly, it was the crucible of her children's health issues that pushed this mother beyond her fears to dig a little deeper and discover a pathway of health and blessing for her family. Keep reading!

Mama Goes Natural:
Plus Bonus Tips & Recipes

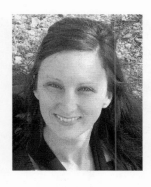

by Kristy Howard, http://www.littlenaturalcottage.com

From Skeptic to Student

Growing up, I *endured* my mother's infatuation with herbs. My siblings and I dutifully took on an air of martyrdom when it came time for yearly cleanses, disgusting-smelling poultices, and healthy green drinks made from bitter-tasting *grass*, no less.

Despite my mom's best efforts, I wasn't the least bit interested in the funny-sounding plants that comprised her world of herbs.

It turns out life eventually rerouted my thinking, but the transformation certainly didn't happen overnight.

I was in my early twenties, married, and about eight months pregnant with my first baby when I visited with a friend who had recently given birth to her tenth baby. I recalled that most of her births had been midwife-assisted, and a strange impulse nearly compelled me to ask her about midwifery and home births. I dismissed the notion before it took root, thinking, *There's no way* I *could ever have a home birth!*

As a new mother, I took the "normal" route with our daughter's birth: an OBGYN, in a hospital, with an epidural. I suffered so many of the side effects of the epidural that I vowed *never again*. Next time, I'd go natural.

I just had no idea how *natural* my life would "go" in the coming years!

I breastfed my daughter, supplementing her with formula in the early weeks while I struggled through worrisome breastfeeding issues. Mostly because I am a stubborn girl, I persevered through our difficult beginning and ended up breastfeeding for sixteen months!

Two-and-a-half years following the birth of our first child, our second daughter was born: at the hospital, without drugs. Her quick but painful birth was my first *real* introduction to the world of "natural"!

Our second daughter's birth came in summer, and my husband and toddler were suffering miserably with allergies, hay fever, and eczema. It didn't take long for me to realize that over-the-counter (and even prescription) medications offered little relief.

One afternoon, my mother (ever the herb lover!) shared with me that household products are often at the root of allergy-related skin conditions. I was desperate to find relief for my husband and daughter, so I delved into my own research.

Curiously, I logged onto the internet and Googled the phrase "how to make your own household cleaners".

To my shock, I discovered a WORLD of information via the internet: bloggers who used cloth diapers, cooked with all sorts of ingredients they called "real food", and even made their own soaps, cleaners, and detergents.

I scoured the web for days on end. Before I knew it, I had bought into a radical new concept: *natural living*.

Mama Goes Natural

Around this time, our newborn daughter came down with a mysterious fever. I had never known an infant to succumb to a fever out of the blue, and I felt a sinking fear settle over me. I called our pediatrician, who instructed me to bring the baby to the clinic right away.

Nearly panicked, I rushed our three-week-old daughter to the office for the doctor.

The prognosis: an ear infection. Easily remedied by the good old pink medicine.

I was relieved and baffled at the same time. Somehow, I felt silly for being so helpless and panicked over something as simple as an ear infection. But how was I to know? And what was I to do about it, anyway? Weren't doctors the ones who were supposed to take care of children?

A feeling of great responsibility washed over me one afternoon as I sat rocking our tiny daughter a few days following our dash to the doctor. As I gazed down at her innocent face, I berated myself for *not really knowing how* to take care of my children's health.

There was the pink antibiotic for the baby, and the prescription cream for my toddler's eczema . . .

What is in that stuff anyway? I wondered. Something deep inside rejected the thought of giving my young children something about which I knew absolutely nothing.

The same doubts welled up inside me at our baby's three-month check-up a few weeks later.

"How often do you see reactions from vaccines?" I asked the pediatrician. He assured me that adverse reactions were rare, thanks to new and improved vaccines.

I glanced doubtfully at our baby and winced as the nurse injected a series of needles into her leg.

That was the last time I took one of our children to the doctor for an antibiotic or vaccine.

I began devouring every book and blog I could find on the topic of natural living and health.

I spent less time at the pharmacy and more time inside the four walls of our health store.

I waged war on white flour, canned soups, and just about every processed food I could think of.

I ditched Pampers, invested in a stash of cloth diapers, and began making my own baby wipes.

I learned all I could about living free of chemicals, preservatives, and pharmaceuticals. My mantra became *If my family needs it, I can probably make it . . . or grow it!*

In May 2008, I gave birth to our third child: at home with a midwife. I was now the mother of two daughters *and* a son, and a veteran natural mama in the eyes of most of my friends and family.

This new lifestyle invigorated me! My thirst for knowledge was nearly insatiable, and the more I learned the more I longed to know. To share my new found love, I launched a blog: *Natural Mama*, a simple description of the woman I was becoming.

My one thorn-in-the-flesh was the chronic issue of ear infections and earaches that plagued our youngest daughter, and now our baby son as well. Why were my little ones suffering with this health issue when I was trying *so hard* to keep them well?

I vowed by the grace of God to never put another drop of antibiotics into my children's mouths, but what was a mother to do? I couldn't very well let them suffer through the pain. It was a long process of learning what *to do*, not just what *not* to do, that kept me a vigilant student of health and herbs.

Early on, I read that *garlic* was a powerful natural antibiotic against ear infections, so garlic oil became my new best friend. I eventually branched out into making my own ear drops with various herbs and essential oils. Despite the many earaches and infections that plagued our children for the first two years of their lives, I never had to resort to antibiotic treatment again. Eventually, I was able to treat earaches *before* they progressed into more painful and hard-to-treat infections.

The Crucible

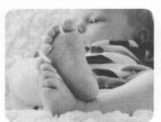

We were blessed with a second son in 2010. As much as I longed to embrace a season of quietness and joy with our new little one, his birth ushered in an intense season of difficulty for our family.

Within days of our son's birth (our second birth at home with a midwife), red flags began to wave regarding his health. Although he nursed ravenously, he could not gain weight. His chubby little arms and legs shriveled into sticks and I cried every time I bathed his thin body. Intuition shouted in my heart that something was very, very wrong.

A trip to the doctor at two weeks post partum proved pointless; the nurse practitioner suggested that he may have colic. I shook my inner head in disgust and took my skinny baby home.

By three months of age, our baby's weight had plateaued at ten pounds, barely up two pounds since birth. A month of countless treks to the clinic to chart his weight revealed zero weight gain.

The doctor eventually offered a prognosis of "failure to thrive" and referred us to the children's hospital 70 miles away, where a series of tests could be run to detect a possible cause for his condition.

My heart sank. By this point, I was nearly convinced that our baby's health issues were related to an unhealthy gut. Although I could not convince the doctor of food allergies, my own research prompted me to remove both milk and gluten products from my diet to prevent possible food allergens from passing to the baby via breast milk.

I wasn't *certain* that food allergies were involved; it was simply a strong hunch.

Our baby's health did not turn around until we sought help through holistic doctors. Over the course of two years of homeopathic treatment, an extremely careful diet, including raw goat's milk supplementation for the baby and a completely allergy-friendly diet for me, and much prayer, our sickly baby boy grew into a thriving toddler.

Interestingly enough, he is our first child who has yet to suffer with an eczema rash or ear infection!

Today, I am the blessed mother of five children. (As of this writing, our third son was born at home just three weeks ago.) As I look back 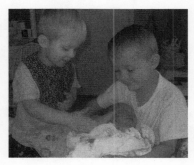 over nearly ten years of motherhood, I thank God for where He has brought me, for the many wonderful resources He has placed into my hands, and for the wise women who have shaped my beliefs and world view. My passion is to empower and encourage other young mothers to "think outside the box" in terms of nurturing their children's health.

Baby Steps for Natural Mothering

If you long to begin this journey of natural mothering but aren't sure how to start, let me take your hand and recommend a few first steps:

1. **Ignore the Naysayers (including yourself)**
2. **Become a Student of Herbs, Whole Foods, and Natural Living**
3. **Find a Mentor (be it a healthy friend, family member, or a favorite blog!)**
4. **Read *Something* About Health Every Single Day**
5. **Don't be Afraid to Put into Practice What You're Learning**
6. **Set Health Goals (know what you want to learn and where you want to go)**
7. **Be Patient With Yourself (it can take years to replace old habits)**

Resources for the Natural Mama

In the past seven or so years of my journey into natural living, I've come across a wealth of helpful resources. Many of the following titles have worked their way into my personal library; I highly recommend the following books:

- *Clean and Green*, by Annie Berthold-Bond
- *The Naturally Clean Home*, by Karyn Siegel-Maier
- *The How-to Herb Book*, by Velma J. Keith and Monteen Gordon
- *Herbal Antibiotics*, by Stephen Harrod Buhner
- *The Green Pharmacy*, by James A. Duke, Ph.DHerbal Remedies for *Children's Health*, Rosemary Gladstar
- *How to Raise a Healthy Child . . . in Spite of Your Doctor*, by Robert S. Mendelsohn, M.D.
- *The Vaccine Book*, by Robert W. Sears, M.D.
- *The Vaccine Guide*, by Randall Neustaedter, OMD
- *Unraveling the Mystery of Autism and Pervasive Developmental Disorder*, by Karyn Seroussi
- *Healing the New Childhood Epidemics: Autism, ADHD, Asthma, and Allergies*, by Kenneth Bock, M.D.
- *Gut and Physycology Syndrome*, by Natasha Campbell-McBride, M.D
- *Making Babies, Book & DVD Series*, by Shoshanna Easling
- *Natural Childbirth the Bradley Way*, by Susan McCutcheon
- *The Natural Healthy Pregnancy, The Naturally Healthy Woman, and Mommy Diagnostics*, by Shonda Parker
- *Nourishing Traditions*, by Sally Fallon

Favorite Remedies

From time to time, friends or family ask me for a specific natural remedy or protocol for sickness. Here are a few favorite remedies I use for my children and recommend to others:

How to Break a Fever

Catnip tea is probably my absolute favorite remedy for bringing down a fever. Unfortunately, most people have never even heard of it! I buy my catnip from Bulk Herb Store and brew it in a tea bag or strainer. In my own experience, two cups of tea usually break a fever within a half-hour. Catnip is mild tasting and is safe for children (even babies). **For young babies,** *do not* **sweeten the tea with honey; use stevia or agave nectar instead.** Catnip blends well with peppermint tea for a tastier drink.

Bear in mind that fever is not a "disease", but a sign that the body is trying to kill off a virus or bacteria. Dr. Robert Mendelsohn's book, *How to Raise a Healthy Child in Spite of Your Doctor*, armed me with a lot of knowledge on this subject.

Sore Throat

For adults and children old enough to swallow capsules: Take 3 to 4 capsules of ground **turmeric**, 3 to 4 times a day. I usually see improvements within a day or two. We've had good results with turmeric for everything from sore throats to earaches and strep throat symptoms. I sometimes open a capsule and sprinkle the powder into soups . . . the spice is similar to curry in taste (although not quite as strong). This is a great way to administer turmeric to small children who can't swallow capsules.

Earaches & Infections

Place 1 drop **warm garlic oil** in each ear; or place a **small garlic clove** in ear and let it sit for 20 to 30 minutes. Garlic kills infection and soothes pain. Both these methods are very effective in relieving pain from earaches and curing ear infections.

Anytime I suspect low immunity or infection, I supplement my children with a quality probiotic. Tummy Tune-up by BeeYoutiful is an excellent product.

Bath Soak for Sick Kiddos

When my children are fighting an illness or are sick, I always treat them to a good "soak". The following bath protocol is effective in drawing out toxins from the body, as well as relaxing and soothing sore little muscles.

- Place about 2 cups Epsom Salt and 1 bottle of Peroxide into a very warm bath (not uncomfortably hot); stir water until salt is completely dissolved. If desired, you can add essential oils for extra health benefits: eucalyptus oil to soothe congestion and open bronchial tubes, or lavender oil to promote relaxation, etc.

Encourage your child to sit and soak in the bath water at least 15 to 20 minutes. While they soak, gently bathe their bodies with the warm water and make it a pleasant, relaxing experience. If the child has a temperature, encourage him or her to drink fluids (herbal teas, lemon water, etc) during the bath to provide maximum hydration.

Cures for Constipation

Constipation is a big deal for a lot of children! Don't fall for the myth that it's okay for your children to have bowel movements infrequently. If he or she is not eliminating two to three times a day, there's your clue that something needs to be done to improve digestive health.

The following steps have been most beneficial in dealing with my children's chronic digestive issues, including constipation:

- **Identify and remove food allergens.** Gluten is especially harmful to gut health when an allergy or sensitivity is present.
- **Supplement with probiotics.** This is a *daily* necessity when constipation is present. You may want to introduce fermented drinks, such as Kefir or Kombucha, into your child's diet.
- As I previously mentioned, **chiropractic adjustments** can be very helpful to encourage regular bowel movements.
- Make sure your child is drinking enough water and getting enough fiber *every day*. Processed foods and junky drinks clog the digestive tract and hinder proper absorption and elimination.

To say I am not the same woman who glibly entered motherhood ten years ago is a gross understatement. *Motherhood radically changed me.* It gave me something to live for, something to fight for.

In many ways, I still fight for my children's health, and so must you, if you are a mother.

Don't believe the myth (as I once did) that your children's health is the responsibility of your pediatrician. Nothing could be further from the truth. No one knows your child as you do, and no one cares for your child more than you.

Knowledge is power, and the knowledge of *how* to care for your children's health will free you from the fear, insecurity, and irresponsibility that plague so many young mothers.

Don't be afraid to trust your intuition!

About Kristy Howard

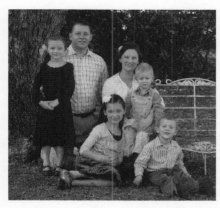

Kristy is a believer in Jesus Christ, a pastor's wife, an aspiring herbalist, and homeschooling mother of five precious blessings. She is passionate about living simply, naturally, and Biblically for the glory of God.

Kristy is the author of The Cottage Mama's DIY Guide, The Cottage Mama Plans Her Menu, and other natural living ebooks. She blogs about health, whole foods, natural living and motherhood at www.LittleNaturalCottage.com

Tell me what you eat, I'll tell you who you are. ~Anthelme Brillat-Savarin

Coming up next! Jill Winger shares the secret to success using natural remedies! Here is a woman who once openly scoffed at people who chose a more natural lifestyle, but found herself drastically changing her tune after having children of her own. Her journey of transformation from a fully conventional life to a modern-day homesteader begins on the next page.

How exactly does a regular gal who grew up in a regular, "standard American" home end up living out on the prairie milking a cow and growing vegetables? Read on to find out . . .

From Intimidated to Empowered

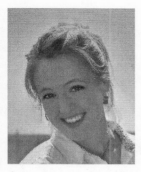

by Jill Winger, http://www.theprairiehomestead.com

Would You Be Scared To Clean A Deep Wound At Home?

I never thought I'd end up being one of *those* people . . . You know, the ones who worry about what chemicals are in their deodorant, or who make "potions" when they are sick instead of going to the doctor, or who don't like to buy food from "normal" grocery stores.

Yet, here I am . . . a soap-making, raw-milk-drinking, essential-oil-loving, mother of two, who makes homemade deodorant, treats my family with natural remedies, and buys everything that I can from the farmer's market.

You see, I started out as fairly "normal." I grew up in a small neighborhood to "normal" parents. We ate typical standard-American fare growing up: soda pop, chips, pasteurized processed cheese product, and the like. When we were sick, we promptly visited the doctor for the expected prescription of antibiotics and went on our way. Natural options or herbal remedies were thought to be a silly waste of time.

As a young adult, I openly scoffed at "health nuts," and I thought it was completely pointless to concern yourself with what was "organic" or "natural." After all, who really had time to worry about such things?

However, I found my perspective changing drastically as soon my first child was born and I realized that I was now responsible for a tiny new life. It only took a bit of research to open my eyes to the dangers of our modern diets and lifestyles and realize it was time to make a change.

The switch didn't happen overnight . . . I began by gradually changing the way I cooked. I shunned my once-beloved canned soups and boxed dinners and slowly learned how to make healthier replacements from scratch. Next, I turned my focus on fats. Initially, I held on to my little boxes of margarine for dear life . . . . I had no doubt that real butter was a healthier option, but I couldn't reconcile the massive difference in price. Fortunately, I eventually gave in and replaced all of the canola oil, shortening, and yes, margarine in my kitchen with healthier options such as coconut oil, olive oil, and butter.

Then came the biggest leap of all—dairy products. I had been reading of the benefits of raw milk, but the laws of our state prevented me from purchasing it. This dilemma resulted in the purchase of two pregnant dairy goats, much to the shock of our friends and family. Our goat adventure eventually led to the purchase of a milk cow. I am now an avid fan of raw milk, as well as homemade yogurt, cheese, and butter.

So there I was, proudly drinking fresh milk, canning my homegrown vegetables, and making all of our food from scratch. Yet when a member of my family became ill, I still felt completely helpless and dependent on the modern medical system.

I will be the first to say that I think physicians and hospitals have their place. If a member of my family has a broken leg or is in a car accident, I am very thankful for the option of having them treated by knowledgeable professionals. However, whenever I visited the doctor for less-serious afflictions, I always ended up leaving the office feeling rather helpless and at the mercy of the system. The doctors I saw had little interest in discussing the health of my body as a whole—they were more interested in writing prescriptions on their little pads of paper. And I couldn't help but feel frustrated that these prescriptions usually only provided relief from symptoms, not from the issue itself.

My desire to be free of this dependence on a flawed system fueled my desire to further educate myself about more natural treatment options that I could administer from home.

Although I've spent numerous hours reading and researching, I still consider myself to be a relative newcomer to the world of natural medicine. So far, I've dabbled in herbs, homemade treatments, and various do-it-yourself skin care products. I've had some great successes, and also made some mistakes. However, I can say one thing without a doubt: The feeling of empowerment and satisfaction that comes with taking charge of your own health is absolutely worth the time and energy it takes to study and research.

Recently, my favorite method of treatment has been essential oils. I'm a skeptic by nature, so it took me quite a long time to become convinced that essential oils were of any value. But once I actually tried them, I was hooked.

The concept of essential oils made much more sense to me once I realized that many of our modern-day pharmaceuticals were originally sourced from nature. For example, the bark of the willow tree was once used as "aspirin," while the modern pain drug, morphine, comes from poppy plants. Unfortunately, science tends to isolate the desired properties of such plants and instead creates synthetic versions, which often result in undesirable side-effects. Conversely, essential oils allow us to benefit from the healing power of plants without many of the issues that arise from modern-day imitations.

I find myself using essential oils on a daily basis to treat everything from heartburn and allergies to asthma and mastitis. I especially love peppermint oil and find it useful for headaches, heartburn, indigestion, or a quick pick-me-up. One of my favorite methods of using essential oils in my home is through a diffuser. I especially like to diffuse anti-bacterial oil blends if someone in my family is fighting a cold or flu.

I've noticed that every time I transition from a conventional approach of life to a more natural practice, I experience some definite moments of doubt. For example, even though I was completely sold on the health benefits of raw milk, I had a slight panic attack the first time I took a sip of our fresh goat's milk. I secretly wondered if I would be doubled-over with food poisoning later that evening. It can be frightening to go against the "facts" that we have been taught our whole life. And at times, you might even wonder if you made a mistake. (I would like to note that after that initial moment of panic, I pushed the fear aside and have now been drinking fresh milk from our own animals for close to three years without a single stomach ache to show for it.)

Another similar instance of doubt happened recently after my husband suffered an accidental dog bite on his hand. Miraculously, only one canine tooth was able to puncture through his thick, leather glove, but the resulting wound was quite deep.

Even though I tried to appear outwardly confident at the time, my mind raced as I attempted to determine the best course of action. I had been using my collection of essential oils to treat milder issues, but nothing as traumatic as a dog bite. I wanted so badly to treat the wound at home, but I was fearful of infection and the possibility of the injury turning into something much more serious. As I debated the options in my mind, it was tempting to load him up in the car and drive him the 40 miles to town to see the doctor, simply so I wouldn't have to try to figure out what to do.

Thankfully, I was able to collect myself and come up with a plan. My main concern was cleaning the bite as thoroughly as possible. We immediately flushed the wound with running water, and then followed that with a splash of hydrogen peroxide.

I chose a selection of essential oils known for their cleansing, anti-bacterial, and healing properties and applied them to the wound before bandaging his hand.

Over the course of that day, I encouraged him to repeatedly come inside so I could remove the bandage, flush it with more running water, and reapply the oils. That evening he soaked his hand in a bowl of warm water and Epsom salts to help further cleanse the wound and draw out any potential infection.

We repeated this protocol over the next several days. We were both amazed to watch this substantial wound heal without any bruising, infection, redness, or swelling. Not a single conventional antibiotic was required throughout the entire process.

Looking back, I am so thankful that we chose to educate ourselves to treat this wound at home. If I had given in to the temptation to rush him to the doctor, not only would have he ended up on potentially damaging prescription antibiotics, but I would have completely missed a valuable learning experience and confidence-booster. It is truly humbling to experience first-hand how equipped our bodies are to heal if we simply support them.

Here are a few of my best tips for starting out with natural remedies:

- **Remember to view the human body as a whole.** Because we as a society are so inundated with the viewpoints of conventional medicine, we are conditioned to think of the different aspects of the body as being completely unrelated to each other. However, the holistic view of healing teaches the exact opposite—Each system of our body can often affect the others in profound ways. (For example, did you know that gum disease can often lead to heart problems?) And don't underestimate the value of good nutrition and adequate rest. These simple measures can often mean the difference between a strong foundation of health or a weak one.

- **Be prepared for episodes of doubt.** As you delve into the world of natural remedies, be prepared to have momentary feelings of doubt, just like I did during our dog bite experience. Don't let these feelings discourage you, but instead, allow them to spur you on to greater understanding and research.
- **Remember that many natural methods of healing have been used for thousands of years.**
  This point is vital to remember when dealing with doubt. Sometimes after I've been questioned about our natural lifestyle by a doctor or well-meaning family member, it's tempting to feel like I'm really "living on the edge" when it comes to my health. However, I always remind myself that people have been using various forms of natural healing for thousands of years, long before hospitals, x-ray machines, or conventional pharmaceuticals were invented. While I am thankful to have access to those technologies if I need them, sometimes the old ways truly are more safe and effective.
- **Be Proactive.** I've found that natural treatments generally work the best when you catch the issue early and treat it aggressively. As we dealt with my husband's dog bite, I made sure to apply the essential oils right away, rather than wait for any infection to take hold.
- **Stay observant**. As I choose to take more responsibility for my own health, as well as the health of my family, it is important to be especially attentive to the signs that our bodies give us. For example, rather than giving my children fever-reducing medications for low-grade temperatures, I prefer to allow their bodies to use the fever to fight the illness. However, you will find me diligently giving liquids and monitoring temperatures numerous times throughout the day while the fever runs its course.
- **Collect a variety of different opinions.** It can be easy to become "hooked" on one website, author, or speaker for all of your information regarding natural living. While there is nothing wrong with having a favorite source, it is wise to listen to a variety of different opinions and thoughts, and then "average" out the results to maintain a well-rounded view.
- **Know when you are in over your head.** There is nothing wrong with admitting that you aren't quite sure what the next course

of action should be when dealing with a health issue. Don't be ashamed to seek help—whether it be from a knowledgeable friend, a trusty reference book, or even the family doctor.

If someone like Jill can make the switch to a healthier, more natural lifestyle, then so can you. It all starts with taking the time to better educate yourself about the options available to you. And remember that the journey must begin with baby steps—one cannot instantaneously go from the standard American lifestyle to making cheese and using natural remedies exclusively. It's a gradual process, but one that definitely can be enjoyed along the way.

About Jill Winger

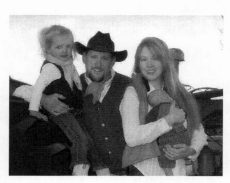

Jill is a lover of Jesus, horses, homespun living, milk cows, natural remedies, and the rural way of life. She lives with her husband, daughter, and son on a 67-acre Wyoming homestead that they share with a variety of farm animals. In her spare time, you'll find her writing on her blog, playing with essential oils, painting old furniture, pulling weeds, and hanging laundry on the clothesline.

The worst thing about medicine is that one kind makes another necessary. ~Elbert Hubbard

Coming up next is a woman who encountered a health condition with one of her daughters that required more than one trip to the doctor. Baffled that her normal remedies were not working, she dug deeper to find natural remedies that would target the specific need and help keep her daughter off medication.

She shares recipes and instructions on how you can easily make these remedies in your own kitchen, and use them for the betterment of your family.

Recipes for Success: Cough Syrup, Lung Formula, Congestion, and Respiratory Sicknesses

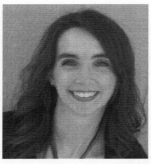

by Jill of Jill's Home Remedies,
http://www.jillshomeremedies.com

I began to use natural remedies when my oldest daughter was only a year old. Being amazed at the effectiveness of natural remedies, I was able to keep my girls out of doctor's offices by simply using natural antibiotics and immune boosters when they were sick. However a day came when I realized that I sometimes needed more than just an immune booster. I will share the symptoms one my daughter had that required trips to the doctor, the doctor's diagnosis' and how I have been able to treat her at home with natural remedies instead of conventional medicine.

A few years ago, one of my daughters began to get coughs easily. These coughs were dry and had a ring to them. She would cough on and on after running hard in a gym, she would cough on and on after playing around dust, and my normal doses of natural medicines were not taking care of her cough as they should. She would get past these coughs, but longer than a few days as she normally did.

During one of her sicknesses, we ended up at the urgent care with a persistent cough that had reached a point where I knew a doctor must be seen. After x-rays were taken, she was diagnosed with pneumonia. While I try to avoid doctor trips if possible, I am thankful for them in serious situations!

I will add here that my daughter did not act or look sick at all when I took her to this urgent care office. She only had a persistent cough that made her eventually throw up mucus. She never ran a fever, lost her appetite or acted lethargic. She was running and playing and eating and happy! I feel confident that this is due to the immune boosters she was taking.

It was only a month later that we were at urgent care again with her persistent coughing, which was not responding to the natural antibiotics/immune boosters. This time she did not have pneumonia, but was diagnosed with asthmatic bronchitis. She was prescribed antibiotics and steroids once again. The doctor said that her recurring cough could be related to asthma and she may in the future need regular medication.

This is of course not something I wanted for her life! Armed with the diagnosis of pneumonia and asthmatic bronchitis, I researched what I could do to help her avoid having to take medication repeatedly for these illnesses, and possibly needing daily medication. It seemed obvious that she did not have strong lungs and they easily got inflamed.

I needed to find remedies that would pull the mucus from her lungs and heal them. I needed foods and herbs that would strengthen her lungs.

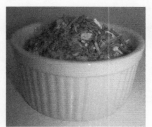

I wanted to avoid future medication, as this problem was recurring often.

The good news is that I found 4 amazing remedies that I have successfully used to help my daughter with her easily inflamed lungs, and have used for the benefit of my whole family! I'm going to share them with you here:

Remedy #1: Lung Formula
{taken from Herbal Home Health Care}

This formula uses the following herbs and is great for treating coughs, asthma, bronchitis, emphysema, and tuberculosis:

- Comfrey
- Marshmallow
- Lobelia
- Chickweed
- Mullein

Combine equal parts of each herb. By combining equal parts, you would use equal measurements of each herb. For instance, a tablespoon of each herb, 1/2 cup of each herb, 1 cup of each herb, etc.—the amount you measure out depends on how much you want to make at once! Mix all of these herbs together in a bag or container.

Let me give you a quick run-down of the herbs and tell you why they are great for the lungs, congestion and coughs!

- Comfrey* heals on contact internally and externally.
- Marshmallow soothes irritated and inflamed mucous membranes.
- Lobelia is a strong relaxant, dilates the bronchial passages and relieves spasms.
- Chickweed acts as a "drawing" herb. It removes toxins and reduces inflammation.
- Mullein loosens and expels mucus. It also calms spasms and reduces swelling in the glandular system.

*Note: There were studies done on comfrey, claiming it unsafe for internal use. In my opinion, further research finds these studies inaccurate. Comfrey has been safely used internally for years and I believe it is safe to take internally for occasional medicinal purposes.

You can crush the herbs and en-capsule them yourself, but my favorite way to use this mixture is in tea form. Add one teaspoon of the herbal mixture to one cup of boiling water. Remove pan from heat, cover with a lid and let the herbs steep for 5-10 minutes. Strain the herbs and drink.

I will say that more than one of my girls has woken up with a croupy cough and constricted breathing. One day of drinking this tea has wiped out the cough and made the breathing normal.

Tea Dosage

Adults drink 1 cup 3 times a day
Children drink half a cup 3 times a day
For my toddler, I place about 1/3 cup of tea in her sippy cup 3 times a day. I fill her cup up with juice so that the tea isn't hot and she readily drinks it.

Another way you can take this mixture is in liquid form. Simply make the herbal mixture into a tincture! You can do this by making either an alcohol or glycerin tincture.

For an alcohol tincture, fill a jar halfway with the dried herbs. Cover the herbs with vodka (I use alcohol for medicinal purposes only) to within an inch of the top of the jar. Keep the jar in a cool, dark place (such as a cabinet). Shake the tincture daily or at least 3-4 times a week.

After 2-4 weeks, strain the herbs, bottle the liquid, and you have a tincture to take!

If you prefer a glycerin tincture, there are 2 ways you can make it:

1. Fill a jar half full with dried herbs. Add boiling water to the herbs, just barely covering, to moisten the herbs. Add food-grade vegetable glycerin to the jar to within one inch of the top of the jar. Let the jar sit for 2-3 weeks {shaking almost daily} and strain the tincture.

2. Another way you can make a glycerin tincture takes only a few days. Place a towel in the bottom of a crockpot and fill your crockpot with water. If you have a shorter crockpot, use 2 pint jars instead of a quart jar so the water comes far enough up on the jars. If you have a taller crockpot, you can use a quart jar. You will fill the jar halfway with the herbs, cover with boiling water and add glycerin to within an inch of the top of the jar, the same as mentioned above. Place the jar in the crockpot and turn it on the lowest setting. I always leave the lid of the crockpot off so the water doesn't get too hot. You do not want the tincture to "cook", you only want to barely heat the herbs. Make sure to add more water to the crockpot each day to keep it full. You can also set the jar on a slightly warm place on a wood stove. After 2-3 days, strain the herbs and store your tincture!

Why add heat to glycerin tinctures? Many people prefer this method because glycerin does not extract herbal properties as well as alcohol, and a little low heat will help it do a better job!

Tincture Dosage

Administer 15-20 drops for adults and about 10 drops for children 3 times a day.

Remedy #2: Homemade Cough Syrup

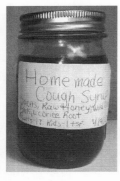

Another remedy I keep on hand is homemade cough syrup. Have you ever looked at the ingredients in over-the-counter cough syrup? According to www.rxlist.com, some of the *common* side effects of children's cough medicine can include: drowsiness, mild dizziness, blurred vision, dry mouth, nausea, stomach pain, constipation, problems with memory, problems with concentration, restlessness, excitability. I also know of a family in my town, who lost a child due to the ingredients in the cough medicine they were administering.

Giving my family natural, effective remedies with safe ingredients whenever possible is very important to me!

Recipe for Homemade Cough Syrup:
(taken from Herbal Home Health Care)

Ingredients:

- Onion
- Raw Honey
- Optional: Add one tablespoon of licorice root and one tablespoon of wild cherry bark. These herbs help to make the cough syrup even more effective, but it is not necessary. I have these herbs on hand, so I add them to my syrup, but the onions and raw honey work great by themselves too!

Directions:

Cut the onion into a double broiler. If you don't have a double broiler, just place a smaller pan over a larger one! You do not want to "cook" this mixture on direct heat as this will kill too many beneficial properties. Cover the onion with raw honey, at least 1/2 inch above the onion.

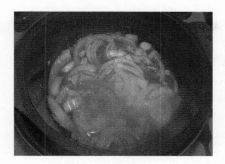

Cover the pan with a lid and slowly heat the mixture on low heat until the onions become translucent. Remember that is very important that you not simmer or boil this mixture. When I fix my syrup, the mixture never has any bubbles in it at all—it just slowly heats and infuses the onions with the honey.

In my experience, it takes about 3 hours for the onions to change and have a translucent look. Strain the honey from the onions and store the syrup in a jar. The syrup will stay good in the refrigerator for 3 months.

Note: One large onion covered in honey yields about a pint of syrup.

If you are concerned about the taste of the onions, it is well masked by the honey. My girls have no problem taking this syrup (not even my pickiest medicine taker), and the baby will beg for some if she sees it! My secret is to not tell my girls what is in the syrup. If I said "onions", they would balk! But if I call it "honey syrup", they take it no problem!

Why onions and raw honey? Onions have natural antibiotic, anti-inflammatory and diuretic properties. Raw honey has antibacterial and antibiotic properties. When combined, these two foods make an excellent, effective syrup!

There are a few things I really like about this syrup:

- It saves a lot of money to make my own!
- It is so much safer to use than over-the-counter cough syrups.
- It can be taken often for frequent, persistent coughs whereas over the counter syrups can only be taken every few hours.
- It works better for coughs and congestion than any syrup I have ever used!

Dosage:

Adults—1 Tbsp
Children—1 tsp.

This syrup can be taken up to every 15 minutes as needed. For bad coughs, allow the syrup to slowly trickle down the throat.

When my girls have an occasional cough or mild congestion, I give them this syrup 3-4 times a day. Most of the time their cough will lessen to a very occasional cough after a few days and I then only give 1 or 2 doses. I typically administer this for a week to ten days total.

For my daughter with more susceptible lung problems, when she begins her constant dry coughing, I give her a teaspoon of cough syrup every fifteen minutes for an hour or two until her cough is lessening. I am always surprised and pleased at how well this helps her! I then give her the cough syrup 3 or 4 times a day until it is gone.

Sometimes I combine both remedies (the lung formula and the cough syrup), administering both throughout the day; sometimes I only use one remedy. I watch for signs and use motherly instinct as to what my girls need for each respiratory sickness.

Remedy #3: Onion Poultice

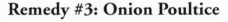

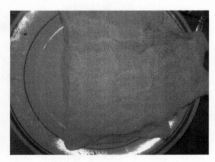

Because onions are so good for the lungs and congestion, making a poultice and applying it to the chest is very effective in breaking up the congestion. More than once I've added this onion poultice to the routine of fighting coughs and congestion.

To make an onion poultice:

- Slice onion (use your judgment on how much you need; it depends on the size of the patient's chest).
- Lightly sauté the onion in a little water for just a few minutes until soft and slimy but NOT browned. I like to get the onion juices flowing and warm, but "cooking" the onions will kill the beneficial properties and make the poultice less effective.
- Place the onions in the center of a towel and fold the sides of the towel over the onion burrito-style as shown above.

You can also roll the onions in the material first and pour hot water over it to release the properties. You would not need to sauté the onions if you use this method. Always be sure that the poultice is very warm but not so hot that it will burn the skin.

Rub olive oil thinly over the patient's chest (to help prevent irritation) and place the poultice on the chest. Cover the poultice with a towel and cover the patient with a blanket to help keep the poultice warm. I typically leave this poultice on all day or all night to let it do its decongestant work!

Remedy #4: Eucalyptus Essential Oil

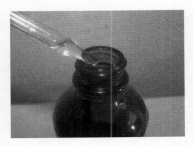

Eucalyptus essential oil is "essential" to keep on hand because it is so helpful in treating colds and respiratory sicknesses! This oil loosens phlegm and reduces mucus membrane inflammation and has many other benefits as well.

There are 4 ways I like to use this oil for congestion and respiratory ailments:

1. Place the oil in a humidifier and place the humidifier next to the patient.
2. Place 5-10 drops of the oil in a full, hot bath.
3. Prepare a steam inhalation. Place a pan on a table and fill it with 6 cups of boiling water. Add 2 drops of the oil in the water, hang head over the pan, covering the head with a towel. Keep face at a safe distance, keep eyes closed and breathe the vapor in for about 10 minutes, taking breaks if needed.

4. Place a few drops of oil on a washcloth and breathe in the vapors for several minutes, not allowing the oil to actually touch the skin.

These remedies have been such a life-saver for my family! I am so thankful I found foods and herbs that target the lungs and can help us avoid more medication. Being on medication myself for 6 years as a teenager and on into adulthood has resulted in many health problems for me. I have been working to remedy my health problems for a while now since I discovered natural remedies. While I do believe medication may be necessary at times for life-threatening situations, I am thankful for the foods and herbs God has given us to use so we can avoid medication whenever possible. It is a great fulfillment to me if I can help my family and others live a healthier life by using natural means.

I encourage you to try these effective, easy remedies the next time you encounter a respiratory illness. You will discover through experience that these amazing foods and herbs are very effective indeed!

About Jill

Jill is a child of God, a wife, and a homeschool mom of 4. As a certified family herbalist, her passions include reading and researching health and home remedies, and sharing with others the knowledge she gains. You can find her blogging at Jill's Home Remedies and connect with her on Facebook, Twitter and Pinterest.

Medicines are not meat to live by.

~German Proverb

We've all had our fair share of fevers, some worse than others. When one pops up, we almost enter into a state of panic, and depending on how high the number reads, we almost forget how to bring it down. This next chapter focuses on why fevers are not the enemy, how they can be controlled, and what their purpose is. Learn how Sara keeps her family thriving naturally . . . with and without fevers!

Fighting a Fever? Think Again

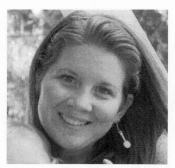

by Sara Shay, http://www.YourThrivingFamily.com

Having a plan in place before you find yourself combating your child's fever can help alleviate their illness as well as save your marriage.

One of the biggest hurdles I have faced in our family's road to more natural living is my husband. Coming from a different background, he had his own misconceptions and myths about fevers. But having an already agreed upon course of action in place can put both our nerves to rest while keeping our children's health our top priority.

Fevers

My foundations in how I go about our family's health began, as early as I can remember, when I was five. My mom has had scoliosis since she was young. I have countless memories of playing with plastic toy animals, while hearing cracks and pops overhead. I loved playing under the chiropractic table!

When we moved to San Diego, our new chiropractor would adjust my brother and I for free. He soon became our first stop if anything was amiss. I also went through a period of having a lot of ear infections; they were most always relieved in less than two days by him applying ball bearings on pressure points. He even diagnosed—to the emergency room doctor's surprise—my brother's appendicitis.

We still received the occasional antibiotics and fever reducers. As well as sprite/coke, chicken soup (from a can) and cinnamon toast when we were sick. I do remember the occasional homeopathic balls as well, but it wasn't what we would typically consider "natural" medicine nowadays. When I was at a point of taking care of my own health a little more, I didn't particularly like the idea of OTC drugs.

It made a whole lot of sense to me, that if there were **things we could do to and for the outside of our bodies, we should do it, rather than adding man-made things to the inside of our bodies**. Once I became pregnant, I immediately was much more aware that my body was not my own. At all costs I tried to not take any drugs—though I was still only equipped with the more conventional alternatives.

I had my first baby naturally and it wasn't till eight months that we dealt with our first real sickness—the croup. If you've been around it, you know how scary the labored, raspy breathing can be. We got through it with over the phone help from my mom. Months later when our little girl had fevers that Tylenol couldn't bring down, we did what most first-time parents do when their child is sick over the weekend—we rushed off to the ER.

The first thing they wanted to do—because she had no other apparent symptoms—was to put a catheter in our little one-year-old. This happened twice. Both times we chose to wait it out. Both times they administered a different form of fever reducer and within twenty minutes she was her happy, rambunctious self again.

A turning point in the outlook on our children's health was when we decided not give our second child the typical immunizations after birth. We had previously not been very happy with all the required pre-school "immunizations" that were given to our daughter. This one was born in a birthing center, on a birthing stool and was a healthy 23 ¼ inch, 8 pound 13 ounce little man. He nursed well, we were home seven hours after he was born and were both able to sleep for six hours. That's unheard of in a hospital birth!

A nurse was sent to our home two days later to check up on our baby, and we were instructed to go to the pediatrician within the first week. He is now over 3 ½-years-old and has been to the doctor only once for sickness. In retrospect I wouldn't do again, but it was close to the weekend and I didn't want to end up in urgent care. We've gone to only a handful of "well" visits. And our youngest, now almost one-year-old, has never seen a pediatrician.

And I will tell you why!

Firstly, we now have three kids. I am past the over-reacting. We've dealt with most of it before. And I am much more proactive in learning about our bodies and how to care for my children myself. The internet, mom blogs and a wealth of information is literally at my fingertips. Now, with smart phones I can cuddle and nurse my little guy while researching the best and various ways to help him.

How to treat fevers, or rather, to give medicine or not, has always been a hot button between my husband and me. My intuition has always told me to let the fever do the work. **God created our body to be able to heal itself**—with proper care and nourishment. We shouldn't have to medicate with every fluctuation of our bodies.

Our position on fevers has taken us almost seven years of parenting to reach. This is probably because we've only had to wade through less than ten incidents of any noticeable fever. And of course in the busyness of being a mom, the only time I devoted to any significant time to research fevers, was when we were in the midst of one.

I believe the struggle between my husband and I is rooted in him witnessing his younger brother have a seizure associated with a fever. This has made him super sensitive when our children have a fever. I hear, "you're going to cook their brains!" He is quick to want to medicate. He also, being the bread-winner, sees our children in the evening—when their sickness seems the worst. They may have been playing normally with a fever all day long, but come night they often have a hard time sleeping.

Each time a fever arises we have a discussion. A HEATED discussion. Ultimately, I know he puts his trust in me to take care of the children. After all, I am the one with them all day and the one with the time to educate myself. But of course I still want us to be on the same page, for him not to have to trust, but actually agree with my methods.

The hurdle for most natural remedies is that you have to stay on top of things and they sometimes take a while to work. **Being consistent and starting treatment immediately is key**. I've warded off quite a few ear infections at three in the morning by being prepared. But for the vast majority of the immediate gratification culture, we get trigger happy with the sticky pink stuff.

Most parents have come to associate fevers with being a horrible thing. They work to make the fever go away, checking for temperature at regular intervals. A few years ago I was surprised to find that even the Mayo Clinic and the American Medical Association caution against lowering fevers.

The way that we treat fevers around here is pretty simple—we don't treat the fever. I take care of the little one carrying the fever. The severity of the fever doesn't necessarily equate to the severity of the sickness. We look at our children's behavior, how they feel and how they act. I'm not going to send them back to school fever-free if they still feel bad, am I?

Knowledge is Power

We talk to our kids about their body and how it works. They have a war going on inside and we have to do all we can to help them win the war as fast as they can. **This really helps with them being willing to do, and ingest, things they don't particularly want to**. Knowing what they are doing and why gives them strength. This also gives them a sense of control in the midst of the chaos they feel being sick.

A Little R&R

Our bodies can't heal if we don't allow them rest. So, on sick days the kids get a lot of reading and more movie time than usual. Even the big kid gets a mandatory nap time, whether she thinks she needs it or not, and she usually *does* end up falling asleep!

Cuddle time is always big, and touch is an important factor in healing. Sequestering them to their beds seems cruel, so I don't do it. Whether I get sick or not, we all get better faster if my kids get lots of love from Mama.

We also have special "treats" for sick days. Maybe they have some favorite jammies or socks (or even some new ones I have tucked away). **Keeping fresh air in the house helps everyone comfortable**. I spray the rooms and put cotton balls into the vents with a few drops of essential oil to purify the air.

We also take **warm baths with Epsom salts and a variety of essential oils**—depending on the other symptoms. It is important for the bath to be warm. If it is cool, the fever may go even higher to compensate for the body cooling down.

The bath itself helps to relieve tension. The salts pull toxins out of the body and help with the achiness that come with fever. I also add a little melaleuca and eucalyptus oil for purification and some lavender oil to relax and calm.

Hydration

If there is one thing everyone knows about fevers, it is to drink lots of liquids—so of course we do **lots of water**. We also **eliminate dairy**, which is harder to digest and creates mucus—something we usually battle when sick.

For the baby, we do as much **breastfeeding** as he wants. If I have been sick too, this means he is getting the immunities that I have built up as well. I have also pumped and given milk to the older kids, in the form of Chocolate Mama Milk. It may be a little taboo, but think about it—isn't weirder to give your kids milk from another species?

Homemade broth, if they will drink it, will help with supporting their immune system, as well as providing more liquids. Skip store bought broths. The benefits are lacking in the mass produced versions. They merely provide flavoring. The typical kid generally isn't willing to drink broth, so easily digestible foods cooked in or with the broth are a good second best. And instead of those electrolyte drinks, look at my next option.

Probiotics. No, I'm not talking yogurt, but **kefir or kombucha**. Both of these you can make at home very inexpensively and are things a normal child will drink. It helps for them to know that this will not only hydrate, but helps all those "good buggies" fight the "bad buggies." I use straight kefir water cut with about a quarter juice for a bit of flavor—the kids love it.

Raw honey is a great treat to give kids when they are sick. Just remember that babies under one year of age, shouldn't have this. Whether it is on a spoon for them to suck on, or on toast sprinkled with cinnamon, it does its job. Raw honey (not filtered and pasteurized honey) can calm an upset stomach, contains many vitamins, minerals, amino acids and enzymes—thus helping your immune system—is anti-viral, anti-bacterial, and anti-fungal, and soothes sore throats to boot!

Topically

Peppermint oil, because of its super cooling effect, is a favorite of mine. I rub a few drops mixed with coconut oil, into the soles of my children's feet before bed. The first time I did this I put some on my son's chest thinking it would relieve it even more. It sure did—he was so cold! Poor little guy, lesson learned by this mama—so don't make that mistake yourself.

There are some other things with garlic, egg whites, and onions you can look up. Personally I haven't tried these yet. I've included some sites that I have referenced for more info—because there is way too much for just one chapter!

Most of the time a fever is not all we are dealing with. It is usually accompanied by a sore throat, runny nose or upset stomach. So these methods, along with things to alleviate the other symptoms are done in tandem.

Getting back to my husband and his preference for fever reducers . . . my chiropractor helped me out on this one. Sometimes it is hard for our spouse to actually hear the truth of what we are saying, much like our children. I know my husband respects our chiropractor, and him having children around the age of ours, helps as well.

This is the deal he and his wife have . . . They treat fevers naturally, to a certain point. As long as the child is acting normal they let it be. But once the fever reaches a certain temperature and the child seems lethargic, they will use an OTC medication.

While this doesn't meet my ideal, having an agreement like this brings peace to our marriage—and thus the house. And when we aren't feeling that great, peace is a pretty important thing!

If you are at that turn in your journey, I just recommend for you to read, read, read. Then try, try, try. If it sounds weird, but it won't hurt your family, try it out. Every little body is different and is going to react differently to each method of healing.

Stock your medicine cabinet with some salts, a few key essential oils and some basic homeopathic tablets, which you should be able to find at your local health food store or online. Educate you children as you are learning more. Make sure your husband is on board, or at least willing to let you try. And most of all, acting quickly on symptoms will ensure shorter healing time.

Sources:

http://www.mayoclinic.com/health/febrile-seizure/DS00346

http://www.nlm.nih.gov/medlineplus/ency/article/000980.htm

http://www.youtube.com/watch?feature=player_embedded&v=N1vZ9m1DES0

http://www.loyolamedicine.org/newswire/features/fever-might-be-your-childs-friend

http://jama.jamanetwork.com/article.aspx?articleid=198355

http://www.naturalmedicinemom.com/how-do-we-best-treat-fevers/

http://naturalhealthezine.com/what-are-the-health-benefits-of-raw-honey/

http://www.mommypotamus.com/natural-remedies-for-a-fever/#

http://creativechristianmama.com/why-i-dont-lower-fevers-part-one/

http://www.modernalternativemama.com/blog/2011/2/26/fevers-good-or-bad.html

I encourage you to check out some of the links for more in depth care of fevers. Always, do your own research and try not to get it all from one source.

Try a few of the easiest out first—those that you can have on hand at a moment's notice. See what works for your family, because every kid is different. And most of all, make sure you have a plan of action in place so that both parents are ready for what may be in store.

About Sara Shay

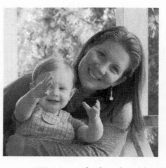

Sara is a full-time mama to three beautiful, sweet & mischievous blessings. And wife of eight years to a man with an amazing heart for working with the youth. She is a Homemaker, gardener, chicken-raiser, doula, and an adjunct & Theatre Tech at a Christian University. Using God as her foundation, she writes about family, food, marriage, children, miscarriage, and pregnancy on her blog—YourThrivingFamily. com Writing helps her hash out a balance between health and reality in the modern world. THRIVING is the goal, not merely surviving life on earth.

Poisons and medicine are oftentimes the same substance given with different intents.

~Peter Mere Latham

Are you scratching your head? If so, be sure to read the next chapter to learn how Kelly Moeggenborg got rid of her children's head lice with natural tools! She trusted her instincts and didn't cave into the "normal" treatments of harsh and harmful chemicals.

Did Someone Just Say 'LICE?' My Tips To Getting Rid of Nits Naturally

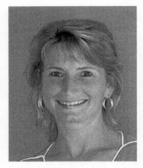

by Kelly Moeggenborg, http://kellythekitchenkop.com

Do you fear your kids coming home with head lice? Do you wonder how to get rid of head lice naturally, without having to use those dangerous chemicals? Fear no more, I've got you covered. I fought head lice and won!

I've always feared the day that lice would make its first appearance in our home. The horror stories of putting everything you've touched into garbage bags for three weeks and covering your child's head with chemicals and cleaning your whole house bottom to top, UGH, I just didn't want to fight that battle! But guess what? I did it. And we survived.

Are you scratching your head yet?

I am, too. Get used to it, it happens whenever you think about lice, but don't worry, that doesn't mean you have it. Not always anyway . . .

Some may wonder why I'm so open on my blog and why I'd tell the world that we recently had lice at our house? Well there are a couple of reasons. First of all, most people know that head lice can come home on anyone, there's no rhyme or reason to it. Also, while I may not personally know most of my readers, call me crazy, but I do think of them as my friends, and I want to offer *help* in case the same thing happens at your house.

So here's what happened to us:

Our daughter had been scratching her head, so of course I looked her over because one of my biggest (non-life-threatening) fears has always been dealing with lice, since I've heard what an unbelievable nightmare it is.

But I didn't see anything. So at first I thought it was bug bites from one late-night playing outside on a warm fall weekend. Then I thought it was the different shampoo she'd been using. When it kept up, I took her to my friend, Patti, who cuts our hair. That's when she found them! AHHHHHHH!!!!! You can see the video at my blog, it's really sick to watch (To find it easily, just Google "Kitchen Kop Lice").

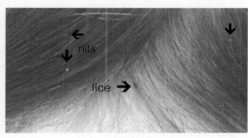

It's terrible to see actual *bugs* in your child's hair! Patti was great and calmed me down. "It's OK, the same thing happened to us when my daughter was little. I didn't see anything for a few days and then there they were! And I'm a hair stylist! *You can handle this . . .*" She also showed me that nits are actually stuck on the strands of hair, whereas dandruff or conditioner that wasn't rinsed out well or whatever just falls off—that's how you know if it's lice nits or not.

I quickly regained some perspective, and knew that there were *much* worse things to deal with in life than lice.

So off we went to the drug store. I bought those nasty expensive chemical lice kits, not for the chemicals, but because that's the only way you could buy the dumb combs. At that point I had no intention of using the poison on my daughter's head.

I called my husband, Kent, and told him that I knew how to treat her hair, because I had an earlier post on my blog full of great info in the comments about what worked for my readers, but I was freaked out about how much cleaning we'd be doing all weekend! By the time I got home he'd been Googling and found an article debating whether cleaning everything from top to bottom really helps, and he thought it would help me to chill out. I said, "Kent, whether or not that site is right, I'm not going to *not* do everything to the house and our bedding, etc., that I've heard we need to do for *years,* just based on one website." I figured better safe than sorry so we didn't have to go through all of this again in a couple weeks!

Here's What We Did to Get Rid of Head Lice Naturally

Based on information from my previous post on lice, advice from friends who have gone through this, and more reading on websites, we took the following steps . . .

- As soon as we got home, I had our daughter get into the shower, as hot as she could stand it.
- Meanwhile, I asked Kent to strip all the beds, grab any towels, coats, or sweatshirts that might be lying around, and get them all into the laundry. HOT water. HOT dryer. Some things we put into a HOT dryer without washing, like pillows without pillowcases, decorative pillows on the couch, stuffed animals, or blankets that had just been washed the day before. Everyone says that 15 minutes in a hot dryer will kill the nits, so I did 45 minutes to be sure.
- We got ALL our hairbrushes and combs and put them into the HOT dishwasher.
- I asked our oldest son, Kal, to start vacuuming the carpets.
- While they were doing that, I started mixing up my lice potion: first I melted about 1/3 cup **virgin coconut oil** gently (not too hot, I wanted all the beneficial stuff still intact), and then added about 1/3 cup **olive oil** and about 12 drops of tea tree oil (from the health food store, which I'd already had on hand, thankfully). Friends have said they just used olive oil and had good luck, but I'd read many good things about coconut oil and tea tree oil, too, so I wanted to be sure!

Once she was out of the shower, I got her onto the kitchen stool and went to work with the combing. I had a couple different combs sitting in some HOT (almost boiling) water in a cup, using one comb at a time, and then dropping it into the hot water and using the other comb for a while. Each time there would be bugs and nits floating in the water, ewwwww! So I changed the water a few times, obviously. I kept going, carefully working through each section of hair, until I couldn't find any more little nasties. This took well over an hour, and she was such a trooper, and was throughout the whole ordeal! According to an article I read, **the key is in the comb**. This is the most important part of treatment (They recommend the metal combs, which I did end up getting, but the cheap plastic ones worked well too, in my opinion).

Then I saturated her hair in the lice potion and covered it with a plastic shower cap; she slept this way for a few nights.

By now I was scratching and decided to treat myself, too, just to be sure. I checked Kent and the boys and they were all good. Although I might have found a nit in Kal's hair, probably not but we were all paranoid, so he asked me to shave him almost bald just to be sure, and I was tempted to do that with all of us!

I called her teacher and asked her to email the class, hoping parents would all check heads and make sure no one came in with it on Monday, so we didn't start the cycle all over again.

I also called her friend's Moms that she'd been with recently, just because it was the right thing to do. Of course they were all cool about it.

Over the weekend (thankfully all this went down on a Friday after school), I washed bedding one more time, and threw a bunch more stuff into the dryer here and there—the dryer ran most of the weekend. I also kept putting brushes and combs into the dishwasher over and over because I was combing through her hair a LOT to make sure I didn't see any nits.

Every time we washed and dried her hair (and mine), we used high heat on the blow dryer, and actually I'll never use cool or warm setting again! My friends who dealt with lice recently swear by this as a good preventative since the lice/eggs hate the heat.

One thing I probably should've done, but didn't think of it again until now, is vacuum out the van where she sits.

Each morning there were fewer and fewer nits in her hair, and by Monday morning I didn't see any. I called the school and they said that the school nurse has to check to be sure, so we met her in the office. Heck if she didn't find TWO more nits. I was feeling discouraged and asked her what she suggested. She didn't pressure me even a little, but just said sweetly, "If it was me, I'd just do *one* of those chemical treatments."

My heart sank

I *really* didn't want to put that junk on her head. I've heard for years how dangerous it is. But she couldn't keep missing school either and I couldn't keep the dryer running *forever*, right? And you should've seen my piles of laundry!

I went to the store and got the "name brand" poison, which was even more expensive, thinking that if I was only giving her one treatment, I may as well take the best shot at it, and this came with better combs, too. I called some close friends, who are also freaks about chemicals like I am, and they were great. They gave me some more good ideas ("Did you try the natural products at the health food store yet? And be sure to ask them for advice, those people know a lot about treating stuff naturally!"), and they also reassured me by saying, "If you have to, you have to, don't beat yourself up over it. Just give her loads of healthy fats and big doses of the fermented cod liver oil to build up her immune system to fight off any of the toxins."

So the chemicals stared at me all day long

I didn't know what to do. I so badly didn't want to put that stuff on her head (especially after looking over those inserts!), but also couldn't stand the thought of going through all this a few more days or weeks, either—I'd read about those who have it keep coming back over and over again! I prayed and Googled and prayed more.

One piece of information I found in my Googling really stood out: these days lice have become resistant to the chemicals in those kits, so the dangerous stuff may not even work! So I might risk my child's health to kill the nits, and there's a very good chance it won't do anything?! Then I knew what to do. I went to the health food store and dropped some more cash. I got a couple of boxed natural remedies and used it on her head that night. The next day we rinsed her head with raw apple cider vinegar, and had her wash her hair with hot water and some Neem oil shampoo and conditioner, since my naturopath friend said Neem was a good lice killer oil.

Once she showered and we blow-dried Tuesday morning, her hair looked great. Linda, the school nurse, looked at it and asked me what I did. I was so excited to tell her and show her the junk I did NOT use.

About the Expense

Here's the thing, I'm not convinced that the $22 bottle of stuff I used really did any more than the lice potion I made up myself. It was the last "oomph" that I needed just to feel better and feel like I was doing all I could, but I do think that between the potion and the combing and the apple cider vinegar and HEAT everywhere, I was pretty much already on top of it all anyway. So if you can be a bit more patient than I was, you could most likely take care of this with a lot less expense than we did.

Prevention!

Hopefully the following plan will prevent this from happening again . . .

I'll be checking her hair more frequently, especially now that I know what I'm looking for. (People say boys get it as much as girls, but I don't care what they say, it just makes sense that short hair is less susceptible, and it sure was in our house.)

When that super expensive Neem shampoo and conditioner above is gone, I'll add a few drops of Neem oil to our regular shampoo.

We'll continue with the high heat blow-drying after every shower.

We'll continue with the high heat in the clothes dryer as long as I'm feeling paranoid, forever probably.

Every now and then I'll throw our brushes and combs into the hot dishwasher.

About the stigma . . .

I was thankful that our daughter wasn't all embarrassed about this. She asked me, "Mom, when it's time to share 'good things' in class, can I share that I'm glad my lice is gone?" Her teacher didn't think that was a good idea, but I thought it was sweet that she wasn't concerned about people knowing. Probably because I was all matter of fact about it. Not that I was laid back about the *bugs* in her hair, this had me freaked out and we combed a *lot* to make sure we got them all, but overall I didn't make a big deal of it and she heard me nonchalantly telling others about it. I've also found out that lice actually prefer clean hair to dirty hair anyway. I have no idea where she got it, maybe church or the store or school, but the school hadn't had a report of it yet this year. However, they did say this: "Most people don't tell."

Hopefully my story helps you relax and know that should lice hit your home, you can handle it, too.

If you're like me and have always feared the day that head lice might make an appearance in your home, take a deep breath. You don't have to expose yourself or your kids to the toxic chemicals in the mainstream lice treatments. I hope my story helps you to relax and know that it can be done, you can get rid of lice naturally. Should one of your kids come home scratching, you can win this battle, too!

About Kelly Moeggenborg

Kelly had a "food transformation" when she discovered the Weston A. Price Foundation in 2004 after a long-time love affair with convenience foods. She began passionately researching how to eat and live better, and on January 1st, 2008 the 'politically incorrect' **Kelly the Kitchen Kop** *blog was born.*

She now enjoys helping others with the knowledge she has gained from her own family's transition to Real Food. In addition to blogging, she also teaches an online class called, 'Real Food for Rookies', and helps individuals become healthier through one-on-one phone or in-person consultations. Check out her e-books: the Real Food Ingredient Guide and the Real Food Party Planning Guide. Kelly lives near Grand Rapids, Michigan with her husband of 25 years and is a Weston Price local co-chapter leader. As if life wasn't crazy enough, she also now homeschools three of their children, and the fourth is in college. ☺

Without proper diet, medicine is of no use.
With proper diet, medicine is of no need.

~Ancient Ayurvedic Proverb

If you know someone with Crohn's Disease, be sure to learn in the next chapter, from Vicky, how carbs in the diet can be a major contributing factor for healing this crazy illness! You will see how diet alone has helped to heal a teenage boy afflicted by this debilitating illness. Researchers now strongly believe that the number of people is growing year by year yet despite many research studies, no one fully understands the disease and a cure has yet to be found. To make things even worse some, if not all, of the drugs prescribed to Crohn's Disease patients are known to have side effects which can often cause further medical problems later on in life. So the discovery that this disease can be controlled just by avoiding certain foods, is almost unbelievable.

When faced with the news that her son's life was threatened by an illness for which there was no cure, a mother with no medical training whatsoever decided to embark on a path of natural healing. This proved to be an excellent approach since now, years later, her son has no symptoms of the disease, in fact his symptoms started to disappear within days of starting this straight-forward diet.

Addressing Crohn's Disease
by Cutting Carbs?

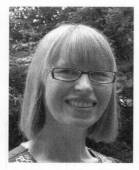

by Vicky, http://glutenfreescdandveggie.blogspot.co.uk

At 15 years of age boys grow and become skinny don't they? I didn't really worry when my son started to become lean because he was actively involved in sports and growing rapidly. He did have dark circles under his eyes but we just thought that this was caused either because he chose to stay up late or it was just a family trait. Looking back, this was probably the first sign that he wasn't well but he never took days off school sick nor had he been ill enough to visit a doctor—until 2005.

On a couple of occasions he complained of lower abdominal pain, which was so intense we visited the doctor. The location of this pain suggested kidney stones but the scan results came back negative.

Early in 2006 we noticed that sometimes he was eating his meals quite slowly, taking a break as he ate because he was suffering a few stomach cramps but these were intermittent. He was always well the following day and anxious to attend school. He was enjoying the rehearsals for his role in the school play.

Shortly afterwards he started to develop large mouth ulcers for which he was prescribed a steroid ointment which actually made no difference. The final suggestion that something was very wrong with his health occurred after a family birthday celebration in early February when I noticed he didn't eat much, not even the birthday cake and this was most unusual. He was clearly suffering from stomach pains and when we returned home his stomach was extremely bloated.

The following day, our family GP examined him and explained that he thought my son might have Crohn's Disease but wasn't displaying all the symptoms. So he was prescribed a PPI, and referred urgently to the local hospital for further blood tests and examination. I had never heard of Crohn's Disease! Later that night I looked it up on the internet, it wasn't a good night.

Those were his symptoms—large mouth ulcers, intermittent stomach pain, dark circles under his eyes and weight loss. The blood tests revealed low albumin, raised CRP and ESR and a low hemoglobin level and these confirmed the doctor's concern. At the end of March we visited the consultant gastroenterologist at the hospital who arranged an endoscopy examination and a barium small bowel meal to try to establish the causes of the symptoms. He also wrote down the types of medication that he may have to prescribe on a small piece of paper.

The endoscopy revealed no evidence of disease much to our relief. The results of the barium meal examination, however, weren't promising. This showed "extensive Crohn's Disease of the terminal ileum including cobblestoning and ulcers with three areas of structuring" but the good news was there was no evidence of fistulous disease. I lie, since this wasn't good news at all! Towards the end of May, the consultant had advised the GP to prescribe Prednisolone at 40mg per day until his next visit to the hospital scheduled for the beginning of June. Unfortunately (or fortunately) we didn't receive any notification of these findings until this appointment. At this point my son was about to take very important Advanced Subsidiary Level examinations.

Prior to this, I had decided to research the medications on the list the consultant had handed over to me at the hospital. The drugs on this list were Prednisolone, Azathioprine and Infliximab and following my investigations, I decided that I would do my utmost to unearth a method that might prevent him from taking these drugs since their side effects were horrendous. Our meeting with the consultant at the beginning of June was the first time I believe I was courageous enough to actually discuss and put forward my point of view regarding this medication. In the past I think I would have been too trusting of the medical practitioners and done exactly as they suggested. However, this was about my son and from within me surfaced a mother's instinct to protect her child.

All the doctors and staff at the clinic were extremely understanding, caring and compassionate. It appeared that my son's illness was one which doctors didn't really seem to fully understand. We agreed that his medication would be delayed until after his examinations and that further blood tests would be taken later in the month. I had three weeks to find a cure!

I trawled through the internet for the possible cause of his disease and for stories of anyone who had managed to recover without having to submit to conventional medication. Two areas of interest emerged. One was Mycobacterium avium subspecies paratuberculosis (MAP) and the other was The Specific Carbohydrate Diet™.

MAP causes Johne's disease in cattle and studies have shown that it can survive pasteurization. Since Johne's Disease is very similar to Crohn's Disease, was this a possible cause of my son's illness? The work of Professor John Hermon-Taylor and his colleagues became of great interest to my husband and I. Since his research suggested that MAP is also present in the streams and rivers of various locations around the UK and my son had been involved in a Duke of Edinburgh Award expedition in one of these locations, drunk water from a stream, sterilizing it only with a tablet which would not kill this bacteria, I believed there was a high probability that he may be suffering the consequences of this action.

I can still remember my elated emotions when I discovered The Specific Carbohydrate Diet™. I had uncovered a possible solution to the problem. I believed that there was a strong possibility that this diet would cure my son's disease and I think I smiled for the first time in days. The principals of The Specific Carbohydrate Diet™ were originally developed by Dr Sydney V. Haas. He discovered that the elimination of certain carbohydrates in the diet improved the symptoms of Celiac Disease. The book, Breaking the Vicious Cycle, was written by Elaine Gottschall following the remarkable recovery of her young daughter from Ulcerative Colitis under the care of Dr Haas.

From the information I had gleaned from various sites on the internet, I immediately began to change my son's diet, cutting out all lactose, sugar, starchy vegetables and grain products. I ordered the book and waited anxiously for it to arrive.

We are a vegetarian family, and at that time I considered that we ate well. The children all had huge appetites but the boys did tend to fill up on bread because like all teenagers they were forever hungry. Since bread was a natural food, I didn't think their diet was particularly bad. Looking back, with the knowledge I've gained over the last seven years, I could have improved their diet dramatically. I bought frozen vegetable burgers and pizzas and there was always a packet of biscuits and crisps in the house. At that time though I rarely went on the internet and I was a busy working Mum with three teenage children, allocating my time between them and constantly ferrying them to their various activities.

By the time the next appointment was due at the hospital, exactly three weeks later, my son was looking much better and hadn't complained once of stomach pains. His blood tests revealed normal hemoglobin, white cell count and inflammatory markers though his iron level was still low. We were elated with this news. However, the consultant did point out that these results did not indicate mucosal healing of his extensive Crohn's disease of the ileum.

The consultant ordered an urgent radiolabelled white cell scan to estimate the activity and prescribed him iron supplements. The supplements contained substances which he was not able to take while on the diet but I was lucky enough to speak to a local midwife who recommended a product which was natural and prescribed to pregnant women. These small sachets of natural, iron rich water from Snowdonia worked wonders! Not only did my son's iron levels return to normal but mine too. Also, I decided to try them myself since five years of taking prescribed supplements on and off hadn't worked for me.

My son started an exercise program to help to boost his immune system alongside the diet which may also have helped him to recover. Due to this incredible healing, he didn't have to attend a white cell scan or any other test that involved "yet another dose of not-inconsiderable amount of radiation in such circumstances." In February 2007 his blood tests were still normal. In fact, the consultant also stated in his notes that, "it is interesting to note that his symptoms have resolved COMPLETELY without any active medical treatment, he has, however, embarked on a modified diet (grain-free, lactose free and rich in probiotics)."

The last seven years have been an extraordinary and remarkable journey not only for my son but for me too. My son continues to follow a vegetarian version of the diet and has completed his University education. I have developed an interest in food and natural cures which some friends and members of my family consider to be quite bizarre. I think most people deem me to be a little over the top where food is concerned. And maybe I am. The food I prepare now is far more nutritious than the food we ate seven years ago and we all eat a mainly grain free, plant based diet.

Nearly everyone I speak to knows of someone who suffers from Crohn's Disease, I didn't realize just how widespread the illness is. The internet is a wonderful resource and I have been fortunate to find others for whom the diet has been successful. I am wholly delighted to have been able to find a "cure" for my son.

When faced with an incurable illness isn't it sometimes worth looking outside the box? Sometimes help is closer than we imagine. I would never have believed that such a simple change in lifestyle could have so much impact. I will be forever grateful to Elaine Gottschall for writing about the diet and for making the "cure" possible for my son.

About Vicky

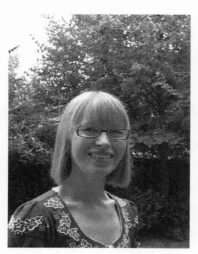

Vicky was born in the fifties and has been happily married for 36 years. She is a mother of three amazingly talented grown-up children. She lives in West Yorkshire, UK, works full time and is very passionate about food. While her primary interest is and always will be her family, she is now the author of a food blog which is mainly aimed at people following a gluten-free diet or The Specific Carbohydrate Diet™.

http://glutenfreescdandveggie.blogspot.co.uk
http://www.facebook.com/GlutenFreeSCD andVeggie

To eat is human.
To digest, divine.

~Mark Twain

Coming up next Stacy Hirsch will share the story of her journey to achieve healthy gut function for herself and her family. Read on to learn how a healthy gut is the foundation for a strong and resilient immune system and how to ensure your child's diet nourishes them for years to come.

Healthy Gut, Healthy Child

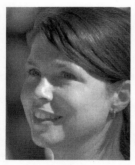

By Stacy S. Hirsch, http://www.TwoTheRoot.com, http://www.stacyhirsch.com

My story with food began many years ago. As a child I suffered from periodic episodes of gall bladder pain. The pain was unpredictable, uncomfortable and difficult to diagnose. My parents tried a few interventions and when nothing worked I learned to love Pepto Bismol. Not because it alleviated the pain, but because it gave me something to do when I felt sick.

By the time I was in college, the painful episodes were occurring more frequently and with more intensity. I continued to seek conventional medicine solutions, but all it had to offer was a tiny pill taken daily for a pain that occurred irregularly. This logic did not make sense to me.

What was different on the days when the pain occurred? Why did it happen at those times? Was it something I was doing?

I said "no" to the medication.

I had more questions and I needed more time to pursue answers. I wanted to know the underlying cause and I didn't want a pharmaceutical band-aid that would only treat the symptoms.

There was a history of gall bladder issues in my family. By the time I was in graduate school, both my mom and grandmother had undergone gall bladder removal surgery for painful symptoms similar to mine. Through my research I was learning so many fascinating things about the body. At the time, I was particularly intrigued by Chinese Medicine and how it made a connection between our emotional health and our physical health. It gave me a whole new perspective on the gall bladder, especially since my earliest memory of stomach pain occurred after my parents' divorce.

From my perspective, gallbladder removal surgery was not an option. It was the wrong direction. It was a short cut with unknown consequences and most likely, broken promises. It might remove the symptom, but without identifying the cause of the pain, new symptoms would follow. Ultimately, I knew it would not take me to where I wanted to go because I wanted an intimate understanding of my body. I believed there was a better, more sustainable way to find relief from the pain I was experiencing. I was determined to change our family story and not continue this particular family tradition.

My intuition directed me to explore the possible link between my symptoms and the food I was eating. My pain almost always appeared within forty-eight hours of consuming a large breakfast, usually an omelet, toast and juice. The omelet was made with cheese, onions and vegetables, the toast was whole wheat with butter and the juice was either fresh squeezed orange or grapefruit. I was certain that one or a combination of these foods was responsible for my symptoms. It was confusing though. How could a whole foods diet be making me ill?

It took me quite a while and a lot of experimenting to realize I had a sensitivity to wheat and gluten. This was fifteen years ago, before gluten sensitivity and celiac had any mainstream recognition. I had always thought of wheat as a soothing comfort food. If my stomach was upset, I was told to eat a piece of toast or crackers. My oma worked in a

German bakery so there were always plenty of cookies, bear claws, cakes and homemade bread. My dad would also make us warm, delicious bowls of Cream of Wheat for breakfast. It took time for me to fully acknowledge and integrate what it would mean to live gluten-free. It also opened a new door to exploring and understanding my overall health.

At that time in my life, it felt like a bold and courageous move, to proclaim I had a gluten-sensitivity. People would roll their eyes and my family and friends treated it as another fad diet. There was little or no support for the idea that common foods, such as, bread, muffins and cereal could make someone ill, but I was highly motivated by my new pain-free existence. I became outspoken. I didn't need research or data. I had a real life experience.

I never looked back.

Trusting my intuition left me feeling empowered. Conventional medicine wanted to fix my pain with a pill, when what I needed was diet modification. We live in a culture where it is more acceptable and supported to take medications to cure disease than to look to our diets and lifestyle. Nutrition is undervalued, overlooked and disregarded as a healing modality and very little attention is focused on the role of healthy digestion and food sensitivities in creating a strong immune system.

Thousands of people die every year from taking prescribed medications that simply mask symptoms and ignore the underlying causes of disease. Understanding our body's dietary nuances offers a safe and effective way to creating lasting health.

Fifteen years after I alleviated my stomach pain by eliminating gluten, conventional medicine is still removing gall bladders, prescribing unnecessary medications and denying that there is a connection between our health and our food. Luckily, people are starting to figure it out and taking their health into their own hands.

Pregnancy and Birth

As my husband and I prepared to have our first child, we were determined, as most parents are, to give our baby the very best start in life. For us, that meant a significant focus on nutrition and immune system support. We both had food sensitivities; he didn't digest dairy well, and in addition to eliminating gluten, I was also no longer eating dairy. This actually helped me remedy years of constipation and bloating. Additionally, I had spent the previous three years recovering from an autoimmune condition. When thinking about our child's health we needed to take into account our combined health history and then plan accordingly.

My personal health journey had taken many twists and turns over the years but I had learned so many important lessons. Prior to pregnancy I completed a training program in nutrition that further underscored the importance of everything I had been learning about gut and immune system health. My husband was beginning his practice as an Integrative Medicine doctor and was seeing first-hand how conditions such as eczema, psoriasis, celiac, allergies and depression, to name a few, were associated with gut and immune system dysfunction. These were all illnesses we wanted to ensure our little one never had to face. We chose to be proactive and work to prevent any future disease.

We had come to learn a lot about our own immunity and its relationship to gut health. It is estimated that approximately 80% of our immune system is located within our gut. The gut, or gastrointestinal tract, is the long tube that begins at our mouth and ends at our anus. A healthy immune response is dependent on having a healthy balance of beneficial bacteria throughout the gut. One way we create and maintain this balance is by eating foods that nourish our gut, such as healthy fats, fermented foods and bone broths, and by avoiding foods that irritate our system or encourage the overgrowth of bad bacteria and yeast.

For optimal gut health and to minimize inflammation in the body, we should all be avoiding foods to which we show sensitivity, as well as unhealthy fats, hydrogenated oils, sugar and refined carbohydrates. Research is now showing that current varieties of wheat actually cause inflammation in everyone's gut, not just a selection of unfortunate, sensitive people.

During my pregnancy, I continued to follow a traditional foods diet that was 99% organic and free of gluten and dairy. I also increased the amount of high quality prebiotics (food for the good bacteria), probiotics and cod liver oil I was taking and included more probiotic rich foods, bone broths and low-mercury seafood in my diet. Probiotics and cod liver oil assist in reducing inflammation in the body, healing the gut lining and preventing allergies. Probiotics ensure that we have plenty of healthy bacteria in the gut. I did everything I knew of to heal my digestive system and support the little life growing inside of me.

I had a healthy and active pregnancy and although our homebirth was foiled by a breech presentation, we created an empowering birth plan that gave us a memorable birth and a beautiful baby. Knowing we would have a cesarean, our birth plan included measures to help mitigate as many of the negative outcomes as possible. One such measure was to refuse antibiotics so that I could maintain the healthy balance of bacteria in my gut. I trusted that my body was strong and that I could fight off any bad bacteria I encountered while in the hospital.

A vaginal birth provides the bacteria that colonizes the baby's gut and makes it strong and impermeable. Having a cesarean birth, the baby misses out on the natural inoculation from Mom and is more likely to be influenced by bacteria from the mother's skin and from the surrounding environment. The next opportunity the baby has to receive a healthy dose of protective probiotics is with breastfeeding.

Breastfeeding

Bacteria from the gut of the mother (probiotics) is carried by the immune system to the breast milk and delivered to the child. Immunoglobulins, cells of the immune system, fight off infection and provide a natural immunity similar to vaccines. Any infection, to which the mother has mounted an immune system reaction, is transferred to the child in the breast milk. This combination of probiotics and immunoglobulins from breast milk is the super food of infants and toddlers.

Studies have shown that breast milk reduces the risk of diseases in infants, such as influenza and respiratory infections, and it decreases the risk of developing type I diabetes or allergies (food and environmental) later in life. Knowing all of the benefits breastfeeding offered, my goal was to breastfeed our daughter until she was at least two years of age.

To my relief, my daughter was a champion breast-feeder and my milk supply was strong. As I breastfed my daughter, I maintained the same gluten and dairy-free diet. Additionally, I stayed away from foods commonly known to upset the tummies of some breastfed babies—onions, garlic, and vegetables in the brassica family. Soon after birth, we also began giving her high-quality probiotics, specifically formulated for infants, and mixed with my breast milk.

Our daughter never suffered from colic, constipation or unexplainable episodes of fussiness or distress. I believe the steps we took to protect, heal, and nourish her gut went a long way in giving us our happy, healthy baby. Her wellness didn't require a pharmaceutical intervention or a visit to the doctor's office. The best medicine was having a well-researched food strategy and understanding healthy gut function.

Solid Food

My daughter began teething at three months and by five months she had her first two teeth. She was physically strong, able to sit up on her own and showed an interest in the food we were eating. All of these signs indicated she was ready to begin solids. We waited for her digestive system to develop a bit more and began offering her solid foods between seven and eight months.

At first, the idea of introducing solids felt a bit overwhelming. I wasn't certain where to begin and my own experience with food sensitivities had left me feeling a bit vulnerable. Avoiding gluten and dairy was an obvious first step given our family's food sensitivities, but we also decided to avoid introducing other grains until after the age of two and then only in moderation and when properly prepared. We skipped the pre-made baby foods entirely and stuck with whole foods we could mash and break into small pieces. I planned our meals around what I was introducing to her so that she could see us eating the same foods. I also maintained a food diary for her so we could watch for any signs of a sensitivity or allergy.

There were a few hiccups in the process. The first time I fed her sweet potato she developed a rash around her mouth. I immediately removed sweet potato from her diet and the rash never reappeared. When we began to feed her fresh foods like celery, apples and grapes we noticed she developed a diaper rash. If we removed these foods the diaper rash disappeared and there was no need for diaper cream which is often toxic. By the age of four she was able to enjoy sweet potato, apples, celery and grapes in moderation.

By removing foods from her diet to which she showed sensitivity, we were giving her gut an opportunity to heal and not creating any new issues. In addition to gluten and dairy, we also made a decision to avoid any food that had a high probability of causing an allergy—corn, soy, peanuts, and shellfish or foods likely to be genetically modified, like canola oil. We also worked with a health professional trained in using applied kinesiology, also known as muscle testing, to identify and clear minor sensitivities, bringing her body into better alignment and balance.

At four years of age, our daughter is vibrant and full of life. She has a healthy immune system and meaningful connection with food. Our entire family still enjoys a gluten-free, dairy-free lifestyle with very few processed foods or snacks. Personally, my health is better than ever and I continue to learn new ways to nourish my family. The most rewarding part is that through my work as a health coach and an advocate for real food, I now have the honor of assisting others to do the same for their families.

So much of who we are as parents depends on how well we know ourselves as individuals. Understanding our personal health journey can give us valuable clues to what our children need to achieve optimal health. A healthy gut is the foundation for a strong and resilient immune response. Undiagnosed food sensitivities can disrupt this balance when left untreated. When we understand how the food we eat affects our bodies we have a powerful tool for helping our children create lasting health.

About Stacy S. Hirsch

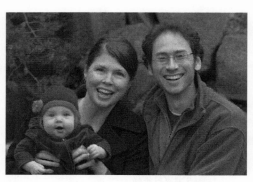

Stacy is co-owner of Beyond Medicine, An Integrative Wellness Clinic, (BeyondMed.com) where she serves as clinic coordinator and as a health coach alongside her husband who practices as an integrative functional medicine physician (DoctorEvan.com).

In 2012, Stacy launched Two the Root, a real food education resource for people seeking a more intimate connection with food. Later this fall she is scheduled to publish two books. Her breakfast cookbook titled, Reinventing Breakfast which combines meal planning ideas with grain-free breakfast recipes that also deliver a healthy dose of vegetables. The second book is a children's picture book titled, "When I Celebrate Food, I Celebrate Me".

Stacy lives in Olympia, Washington with her delightfully curious four-year old, her musical-loving husband and their cat Ava, who never passes on an opportunity to indulge in a warm sauna. Together they enjoy traveling, playing in the garden, cooking and weekend trips to the farmers market.

One of the first duties of the physician is to educate the masses not to take medicine . . . . Soap and water and common sense are the best disinfectants.

~William Osler

Sometimes it's important to seek out a medical opinion, even if you don't intend to treat the diagnosis as a doctor might recommend. That's exactly what the next author did when she was unsure of exactly what she was dealing with, but once she was armed with more information and a proper diagnosis, she chose to use natural remedies and a "wait and see" approach before rushing out to fill that prescription.

It seems that antibiotics are the answer to everything these days, but the times when we really need them should be few and far between. Most of the time, a thorough understanding of the problem and careful treatment with appropriate herbs or remedies will allow us to avoid antibiotics and still achieve excellent results. This is the story of a mom who said "no" to the doctor's antibiotic prescription, and was able to bring healing to a deep skin infection using simple ingredients.

How I Healed My Son's Skin Infection Without Antibiotics

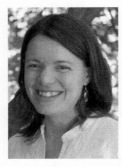

By Stephanie Langford, http://www.KeeperOfTheHome.org

This is a tale of how a mom can take charge of her family's health.

It isn't necessarily meant to read like a "how-to" (although you may find what I share useful), nor is it meant to make some sort of definitive statement about doctors and home remedies and antibiotics (although some may read that into it).

Rather, it is meant to be **a descriptive story of one situation where I used a simple remedy to deal with a health concern that supposedly required medication.**

Here's the story:

For a little while, I had noticed some small bumps on the back of my son's leg. They were unlike anything I had seen before, but didn't seem particularly alarming. As a couple of them grew slightly, I began to be mildly concerned. Baffled, I wondered if they were similar to a pimple or even a manifestation of some sort of inward toxicity, because my son is particularly sensitive to toxins and doesn't handle them well. I tried looking on the internet to figure it out, but finally realized that I just had no idea and it was time to see a doctor when one became infected.

The doctor diagnosed the little bumps as something fairly benign, a type of wart-like virus common to children (passed around in swimming pools, on towels or soft toys, etc.) that is known as "mollescum contagium." **He also confirmed that the redness and pain he was experiencing around one bump was a deep infection**—you could feel that it was a bit hard under the skin, which the doctor said was a pocket filling with infected pus.

The doctor recommended a round of oral antibiotics (which I wanted to avoid if at all possible, as they have very negative effects on digestion and gut flora). **When I specifically asked about topical treatment instead, he told me that it was too deep to treat topically.**

Oh, really?

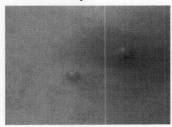

Doctors everywhere, please don't tell me things like that. I take it as a direct challenge. I set out to prove him wrong as soon as I got home.

You can see two of the molluscum in this picture, with the one on the right clearly infected.

How I treated the infection

I chose to treat it with a poultice of raw honey, activated charcoal and a few drops of tea tree oil.

Why I chose my particular arsenal of ingredients from my natural medicine cabinet:

- *Activated charcoal powder.* It draws out toxins extremely well and can eliminate harmful bacteria as well. This that I watched last year came to mind as I considered whether I would use charcoal and how I would do it.
- *Raw honey.* I needed something to make the charcoal into a paste with (otherwise it was just a powdery mess), and I chose raw honey because it also has antibacterial qualities and has been known to help heal other types of infections.
- *Tea tree essential oil.* For its antiseptic and antiviral qualities. I had also found a helpful blog post sharing how one women (and many others in the comments) had used tea tree oil for treating mollescum contagium.

This mixture was a bit goopy and gross looking, and he didn't love the

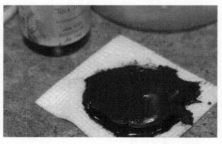

feel of it on his skin, but then again, he didn't like having a painful infection either. I made it clear that I knew he didn't like it, but I really wanted to help the owie on his skin, and he consented, because I guess the owie felt worse than the goopy poultice.

At first, I used gauze pads so that I could cover a larger area, because the infection was spread out beyond the initial site where it began (it was about an inch in diameter). Gradually, I switched over to Band-Aids, once the infected area started to shrink.

Within a day or two, I could see that it was slightly less red and inflamed looking.

Within a few more days, it was definitely smaller in size, and the hard area under the skin was also much smaller. It wasn't causing as much pain anymore (though it was still a bit painful).

The second week, it continued to decrease in pain, redness and size. At this point, I wasn't being quite as on-the-ball with the poultices. I began changing them less often and I moved to just a band-aid with a bit of the mixture, and occasionally, just with a herbal healing salve instead of the black sticky mess that the charcoal made.

We definitely missed a few days, and sometimes he took the Band-Aids or poultice off because they were bugging him (although he was a very good sport overall).

At the 2-3 week point, it looked as though the infection was entirely gone and just a small mark remained where it had been. Now, at the 4 week mark, you can't even tell he had it at all. The skin looks completely healed.

What I Am (and Am Not) Saying Here

I can already hear some of your thoughts, so I'm going to address them proactively:

1. **I am not saying that we should avoid doctors or that their suggestions should necessarily be ignored.** There are times when conventional medical treatment is the right course of action, but

I think it can be helpful to **ask ourselves some good questions before making a decision** for either natural OR conventional treatment. As a matter of fact, I thoroughly appreciated the quick and accurate diagnosis the doctor provided, which I had not been able to figure out on my own.

2. **Antibiotics are not the enemy.** They are overused, abused, and are causing problems as a result of reckless prescription. Much of the time, infections could be treated more naturally or simply be allowed to run their course for a full recovery in a similar period of time. And yet sometimes, antibiotics are invaluable and even life-saving. I'm not opposed to antibiotics. I'm grateful to live in a time and place when they are available for us when we need them. But that's the key word . . . *need.*

3. **Home remedies can, and often do, work as well or better than many prescription/allopathic medications.** They're not something to mess around with, though, particularly if you're not sure what you're doing. I've been studying alternative health and natural remedies for years, and as a result, I feel comfortable treating many of our family's ailments. It's worth noting, though, that before I took this infection on, I had it diagnosed so that I knew clearly what I was dealing with. My husband and I also had a conversation where we agreed that if it didn't show signs of improving within a couple of days (we set a specific date) then we would reconsider filling the prescription for the antibiotics.

This story really is a great example of how a mom can "trust her intuition" and treat a situation without just resorting to the standard medical response. The next time you're faced with something, pause and consider all of your options before simply going along with the conventional advice. Part of our job as moms is to learn to discern when to go with the doctors and when to stick to our guns . . . so trust your gut, mama! You know your family and you are absolutely capable of using natural remedies to help them.

About Stephanie Langford

Stephanie Langford's interest in health and natural living began when she used whole foods and traditional nutrition to bring healing to some health challenges, but it deftly grew into a love for backyard gardening, home remedies and herbs, making homemade beauty and cleaning products, and living more simply and sustainably. She has a passion for sharing ideas and information for homemakers who want to make healthy changes in their homes, and carefully steward all that they've been given.

Stephanie has written three books geared to helping families live more naturally and eat real, whole foods, without being overwhelmed, without going broke and with simple meal planning. She is the creator of Keeper of the Home, and also shares her family's travel tales on EntreFamily Travels.

Our greatness lies not so much in being able to remake the world as being able to remake ourselves.

~Gandhi

Don't miss reading next about how Stacy Karen discarded conventional practices and built her "Delightful Home" by going back to the basics. This mom of three has baby-stepped her way to health and wellness. Her journey began as one of insecurity and uncertainty, but she has now reached a place of confidence in the benefits of natural healing and a mother's intuition. This chapter focuses on the basics of keeping your family healthy and whole and provides tips and recipes for creating your own remedies

No More Vics, Vapo, Vaccines, and Vegetarianism—How I Trusted My Intuition

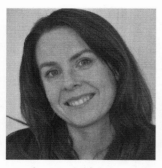

By Stacy Karen, http://www.ADelightfulHome.com

My interest in health started at a young age. Growing up training as a dancer, I spent a lot of time striving to be "healthy," but it had a somewhat ugly undertone. I didn't truly want to be healthy for health's sake. I wanted to be skinny. I wanted to impress the judges and win roles at auditions. I didn't think much about my future self, but rather focused on the here and now.

I believed most of what I heard in mainstream media, tried to eat zero fat, and listened to the advice of magazines and modern medicine.

As I grew in to a young woman, I become more and more unwell. Doctors could not find anything wrong with me, but I felt terrible most of the time. Severe stomach pains and fatigue were common problem.

I was not healthy.

As a new bride, my poor husband worried and fretted over what was wrong with me. I'd be in pain or completely exhausted, for no apparent reason.

This time of frequent discomfort pushed me to search for answers. I never found out exactly what was wrong with me, but as I researched and tried many alternative medicines and herbs, I grew to love the fact that God created so many natural ways to heal the body.

I gave up my 8-year vegetarian/low fat diet, and the color started to return to my cheeks. As I began to eat real food, with good fat, my health started to improve. By the time my first child was born, I had come to feel healthy and whole again.

It was after the birth of my daughter that my interest in natural health grew to new heights. Being in charge of this little life was such a huge responsibility; I wanted to do what was best for her (as most mothers do), but didn't know how.

There were many things during those early days that felt wrong to me. For example, putting petroleum jelly on my baby's face to help with dry skin didn't seem right. I thought the petroleum jelly might contain harmful ingredients, but I wasn't sure which ones, and worried that I was being over-the-top and paranoid. Everyone else was using it. I continued to use products like this on my daughter, even though I felt uneasy about it. Only later did I learn of the dangers of petroleum and find that it was an ingredient in many skin care products, including petroleum jelly. I have now learned to make my own, non-petroleum jelly. It is so quick and easy. The best part is that I can use it without fear or apprehension.

Being very much a rule-follower and people pleaser, bucking the system and learning to say "no," has been difficult. Even though my intuition told me that my intentions were good and right, I was constantly afraid, not just for the health and safety of my children, but also I cared what others would think of me.

When my daughter was born, I thought "good mothers" obeyed all the doctor's orders, kept every well check appointment, and gave their children each and every vaccination on schedule. Since then I have learned that a mother knows her child better than anyone, that a mother has the right to research and question, and is within her right to make requests or refuse certain treatments if she feels it necessary.

My daughter had some sensory issues. Because of this, I felt it necessary to avoid as many chemicals and unnatural medicines, foods, and products as possible. My courage grew because of her.

With a little research and experimentation I've found many simple ways to create natural products for my family. We now use them almost exclusively.

Creating homemade natural body care products and home remedies is not as complicated as one might think. Most of the natural products and remedies I make involve nothing more than measuring, steeping, melting, and pouring. The bonus to creating these products at home is that it usually saves money and also brings a great deal of satisfaction. I can't quite explain the joy I feel when finishing a batch of vapo rub or Echinacea tincture, but I sure wish everyone could experience it!

A pivotal moment happened for me after attending a short seminar by a local naturopath, I came away with scribbled notes, recipes, and excitement. I finally began to feel that home remedies might actually work and that I didn't have to run to the doctor every time my child came down with a cold.

The next time my daughter was sick, I tried out some of my new found knowledge. I will admit to doing so with a little trepidation. I was afraid it might not work or that I'd give her the wrong dosage and harm her in some way, but we made it through just fine.

Around this time I also had the good fortune to meet another mother who was further along the natural living road than me. She talked about the things that worked for her son, explained how some remedies worked and encouraged me along the way. Our interaction was rather brief, but seeing someone in the flesh, living out my ideals, encouraged me.

With each illness, it gets easier to trust my intuition. Seeing remedies in action, healing without the need for harsh antibiotics or lengthy doctor's visits, has reassured me. Educating myself through reading books, doing internet research, attending seminars, and enrolling in a family herbalist course, has also boosted my confidence.

That's not to say we don't go to the doctor on occasion, or that we don't use conventional medicine from time to time. We do. However it is much less often and I feel more empowered to make decisions.

I am only a little way down the road of my natural living journey, and hope to continue growing and learning, gaining more confidence to identify problems, trying new solutions, and passing them on to my children for future generations.

Here are some of my favorite remedies for keeping my family healthy inside and out. Use these recipes to replace un-natural products in your cabinets and care for your children without fear of harm.

Astragalus

- Astragalus is an excellent preventative herb and should be taken prior to the onset of illness. I use Astragalus to help build the immune system.

- Astragalus is thought to be one of the most effective herbs for building the immune system and increasing the body's resistance to disease.
- Besides cold and flu prevention, Astragalus is often used to treat long-term illness or infection such as recurring flu, chronic colds and the Epstein-Barr virus. It is also helpful as a diuretic, digestive aid, and general energy booster.
- Astragalus comes in capsule and tincture form and is easily found at most health food stores. General dosage is about ½ to 1 teaspoon, two or three times a day. Check your particular brand for dosage instructions.
- Astragalus can also be purchased in dried form and added to soups to boost their immune building power.

Homemade Vapo Rub

When my children are congested, I whip up a quick, emergency vapo rub made with olive oil and essential oils.

Instructions:

- Pour 1 ounce of almond or olive oil into a small bowl or cup.
- Add 10 drops total (not each) of eucalyptus, peppermint, or rosemary essential oil (or a mixture of all three, but no more than 10 drops).
- Rub on the chest and back to alleviate coughs and congestion.

Non-petroleum jelly

This is what I use instead of petroleum jelly nowadays. I use non-petroleum jelly to smooth dry patches of skin or provide a protective layer or barrier when needed. It also doubles as a lip gloss.

How to Make Non-Petroleum Jelly

Ingredients

1/8 cup grated beeswax (about 1 ounce)
1/2 cup olive oil

Method

Combine beeswax and oil in a small saucepan. Melt over very low heat or in the top of a double boiler.

Pour into a jar to cool.

Calendula Salve

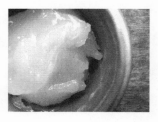

Calendula is highly favored for its skin healing properties. It is also excellent for sensitive skin, making it perfect for using with babies and children.

Making a salve harness the calming and anti-inflammatory powers of this wonderful plant.

Calendula salve is useful in healing many skin problems, such as:

- Rashes (including diaper rash)
- Chapped lips
- Cuts and scrapes
- Dry skin
- Minor burns

In my opinion, the variety of conditions this salve treats, makes it a product all households should have on hand.

How to Make Calendula Salve
Gather the following ingredients and supplies:

1/4 cup dried calendula petals
1/2 cup extra virgin olive oil
1/8 cup grated beeswax or beeswax pastilles
10 drops lavender essential oil (or more if desired, up to 40 drops)
Cheesecloth
Heavy pot
Spoon
Measuring cup
Rubber band
Crockpot

Step One: Place dried calendula petals in a clean jar and pour the olive oil over the top. Close lid tightly and shake to blend. Allow to sit for one to two weeks until the oil turns a golden color.

Step Two: Lay cheesecloth over the top of a glass measuring cup and secure with a rubber band. *Slowly* pour the olive oil through the cheesecloth so the petals are caught on top and the oil goes through into the measuring cup. (I really do mean go slowly. If you proceed too quickly, the oil will run off the sides!)

Step Three: Pour strained oil into a heavy saucepan and turn the heat to low. Add the beeswax and stir occasionally until melted. Add the essential oil and stir to distribute.

Step Four: Pour into a clean container, leaving uncovered until completely cooled.

Step Five: Cap and label. This salve should last for a year.

To use: Rub Calendula Salve on cuts, scraps, rashes, or dry skin a few times a day.

For diaper rash, use after every diaper change.

Lessons Learned Along the Way

Some of the most important lessons I have learned along this journey of health and wellness involve trusting my own abilities as a mother. I have come to understand that I am capable of taking care of my children. Yes, sometimes I need help, and I can't do it all, but I am equipped for the task of raising healthy children and ministering to their needs when they are ill.

I have also learned that a mother has the right to refuse or request specific care for her child; that it is perfectly acceptable to ask questions and seek second opinions.

I've learned that many home remedies are simple and easy to make. Keeping a few supplies on hand along with some basic recipes means I'm prepared for many illnesses when they strike.

And for myself, I've learned that "skinny" does not mean healthy. I'm sad when I think back to the *"me"* I described in the beginning of this chapter. I was a girl who worried more about how the outside looked than the state of my inside. I am thankful to have grown past this and now strive to cultivate a healthy person, mentally, physically, and spiritually.

My journey began in a place of poor health and uncertainty. My path to natural living was paved through self-education and experimentation with home remedies and other natural living practices. Equipping yourself with knowledge and life experience will help bring you confidence and peace.

About Stacy Karen

Stacy is the mother of three children and a minster's wife. She grew up in Australia and moved to the U.S.A to marry her sweetheart. She has a nutritionist certification through Liberation Wellness and is currently studying as a Family Herbalist. Stacy enjoys all things DIY and is often making skin care products, home-cooked meals, or other random projects. She blogs about healthy, natural living at ADelightfulHome.com and has published "Simple Scrubs to Make and Give," a comprehensive guide to making all-natural body scrubs.

Victory is won not in miles but in inches.

Win a little now, hold your ground,
and later, win a little more.

~Louis L'Amour

Up next, read Gina Mooney's amazing story of how she made "Slow" her new "Fast" and how Cha-Cha-Chia Seeds became her new running superfood! From the blog Slow is the New Fast, this mother of 5 will discuss running, her 76 pound weight loss journey and the Amazon Super food that helps her go the distance with her marathon training.

Fat to Fast—How I Changed My Life to Get Off my Couch and Into a 5K in Only 6 Weeks!

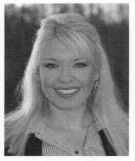

by Gina Mooney, http://www.SlowIsTheNewFast.com

I grew up as an active, healthy child in South Mississippi. Although, my parents always made sure we had wonderful food on the table, the South's way of eating well wasn't always the healthiest way. This really wasn't a problem for me while I was growing up or even as a teenager. After my first child was born, my weight seemed to go back to normal after about 6 months without a lot of extra effort. Fast forward to after the birth of my 4th child.

My pregnancy had gone well until the last month or so when my blood pressure began to get too high and I had to deliver him 2 weeks early. This set this stage for a continuing problem with my blood pressure long after having him. As the months went by after delivery, I began to experience depression and some weight gain. I decided to go to the doctor for help. While there, they noticed that my blood pressure was extremely high. So, I left that day not only on depression medication but also high blood pressure medication. Not only was my blood pressure out of control, so was my weight. At 225 pounds, I stopped stepping on the scale because I couldn't bear to see it anymore.

After my 5th child was born, I had been nursing her and noticing that it was helping me lose a little weight (along with it being extremely beneficial to her). I decided to use this momentum to start making positive changes in my life.

I first began walking around my neighborhood in the evenings. As I became more fit, I started taking the baby and my oldest daughter with me to our local paved walking/biking trail for our walks. As time went on, my daughter would push Zoe while I ran ahead a little ways and then I'd run back and then walk with them more. Looking back, I was doing my own version of the Couch to 5k Program, even though I didn't know it existed.

On February 8, 2010, it was a chilly day and my daughter was sweet enough to watch Zoe at home for me while I went to the trail by myself. As I drove over, a crazy thought kept popping up in my head. I wanted to attempt to run without stopping. The closer I got to my destination, the more excited and nervous I got. I don't know what it was but something inside of me knew that it was time to try. I assured myself that I could always walk if I needed to, stop if I had to, but I was going to at least try. I had no time in mind. It didn't matter about being fast. My goal was to run without stopping to walk.

As the miles ticked away, I began to feel a sense of overwhelming excitement. I felt like a butterfly breaking out of its cocoon! I was a runner! After that day, a fire was lit inside of me and there was no turning back. I'd been reminded that I could do whatever I set my mind to.

Those first steps set me in motion for things I'd never imagined.

I kept training with my mind set on being able to run in a race one day. A little over a month later on March 19, 2010 I ran in my first 5k race. Then, on April 3, 2010, I ran in the Crescent City Classic, which was my first 10k race. During that first year of running I ran several 5k races and also the 10k. I had to deal with shin splints and a stress fracture for 6-8 weeks because of over training. I started back as soon as I was healed and began training again but a little more wisely. I also started slowly adding more mileage to my runs. I realized that I enjoyed going the longer distances and that this might be the type of running that I was meant for.

My longer runs were slower runs and I found myself forgetting that I was exercising and began enjoying the beauty and peacefulness around me. As I continued to bump up my miles, my husband I started decided we'd like to run in a half marathon. So, we began to train for our first one and ran it on January 10, 2011. In April 2011, I had the pleasure of meeting Chris McDougall (author of Born to Run), his trainer Eric Orton and ultra runner, Scott Jurek. Hearing them speak and getting the opportunity to run with them only fanned the flames when we began discussing the possibility of running a marathon.

We began our marathon training in the Fall of 2011 after our racing season was over in May. I ran the Jazz Half Marathon in October with our sights set on the Rock 'n' Roll Marathon New Orleans in March 2012. Unfortunately, a few days after my half marathon, a suffered a horrible fall while out on a training run and broke my arm that required surgery to put in metal plates. Two weeks later, after my stitches were removed, I began training again with a splint on my arm. On March 4, 2012, I crossed the marathon finish line in New Orleans.

Since my journey began, I've lost 76 pounds through running, cross training, making healthy food choices and drinking water. As I drove home that day in February 2010, I would have never dreamed that I would have completed my 2nd marathon on February 24, 2013. More importantly, I've become a healthier version of me and I feel like I can be a better wife and mom. I no longer take medication for blood pressure or depression. I've realized that the best medicine isn't man made but is available to us in the healthy foods we eat.

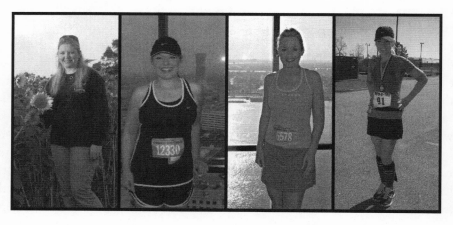

How I Discovered the Power of Chia Seeds

I first heard Chia seeds mentioned when I was reading Christopher McDougall's bestselling book, *Born to Run*. I was just getting fully invested in running and was looking for healthy ways to energize myself and my runs. Before that, the only chia I'd ever heard of was a Chia Pet! Imagine my surprise when I found out how much power was packed into those tiny little seeds! (I was also surprised to find out that they are the actual seeds that grow the Chia Pets, not a distant cousin!) The name Chia actually comes from the Aztec word "chian" which means "oily".

I was very interested to try them for myself so I headed over to our local health food store and bought a bag. In McDougall's book, he describes how chia fresca (chia seeds, water, citrus juice and honey) serve as a "home brewed Red Bull" for the Tarahumara, a tribe of natural super athletes in Mexico who routinely run 50-100 miles at a time.

Chia seeds are rich in antioxidants (more than blueberries), a form of omega—3 fatty acids that don't have to be converted for use in the body (Omega 3s are said to help with hypertension and joint pain)—more than salmon, minerals (more calcium than milk), vitamins, more bran than most bran products and are about 20% protein.

When you soak the seeds for at least 30 minutes, you will notice that the water begins to form a gel-like consistency. Studies have shown that this is the result of the soluble fiber in the seeds. It is also believed that they keep this gel-like texture in the stomach which creates a barrier between carbohydrates and the digestive enzymes that break them down. This slows the conversion of carbohydrates to sugar which means that they can be a natural aid in controlling diabetes (How amazing is that?).

They are also considered to be *hydrophilic*, which means that they can quickly absorb large amounts of water. This was one of the reasons I was so interested in them. These tiny little seeds can hold more than 12 times their weight in water! This makes them ideal for runners or anyone else that's looking to improve their endurance and prolong hydration.

There are so many other amazing facts about these seeds, it's no wonder they are known as "the running food" in Mexican and Native American cultures. Paired with water, they were the main food that Aztec warriors took with them to war. Supposedly, only 1 tablespoon could sustain a person for 24 hours. They were so valued that they were used to pay taxes to the nobility in ancient times. The Aztecs also used them to help with skin condition and to relieve joint pain. Even though they didn't know what we know now, it was obvious that they were aware that this was a very special food.

As I mentioned earlier, I had been reading about the different ways to use them and decided that I wanted to try my hand at making the fresca. I was a little unsure of how I would like it since some of the reviews said it was a little slimy and thick but others remarked that it wasn't difficult at all to drink. I mixed mine up but left out the honey only because I was trying to ease myself into trying something new and, even though I use honey in cooking and for sore throats, I don't always enjoy the taste of it. I left mine for longer than 30 minutes to ensure that they had plenty of time to absorb the water. While the consistency was indeed thick, it didn't bother me at all and the taste was great!

I had read that the seeds would easily take on the flavor that was added to them and it was true. The light lemony taste was refreshing and I actually enjoyed the textured the seeds provided. This drink has become a regular part of my routine when I'm preparing for a long run. My husband has also adopted this drink as part of his pre-run hydration ritual.

Chia Fresca:
1 cup of filtered water
1 tablespoon of chia seeds
2 teaspoons of lemon or lime juice
2 teaspoons of honey

Since then, I've incorporated them into other things I eat. I've added them to cereal, oatmeal and Greek yogurt. They can also be added to bread, granola or muffins.

It's tempting to say that Chia seeds might be nature's perfect food with no gluten, simple sugars or cholesterol and only 137 calories per ounce!

I'm so glad that I found out about them and have incorporated them into my diet. I hope you'll pick some up and see how they work for you!

About Gina Mooney

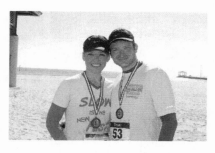

Gina is a 39 yr old stay-at-home mom that struggled with high blood pressure, being overweight and depressed until making the decision to make a change in her health after the birth of her 3 yr old daughter in 2009. By making healthy changes in her diet, drinking water and running, she was able to lose 76 pounds and has just recently completed her 2nd marathon in February 2013.

She now has resolved to pay it forward by encouraging others to become more healthy and active. She was recently featured in a video segment by MSN/Fitbie (Everyday Champions) and was also in the January/February 2013 edition of Women's Running Magazine. Gina is married to Jason and they live in South MS with their 5 children.

A smart mother makes often a better diagnosis than a poor doctor.

~August Bier

Coming up next is the story of a woman who completely overhauled her life, by taking control of her food choices, modifying her day-to-day activities, and ultimately putting her family onto a path toward health. Her journey began with the birth of her first child and as her family has grown, she appreciates more and more the benefits of natural health and healing. Keep reading to learn how a typical American girl went from living a typical American life to improving her health, thus teaching her children good lifestyle choices from an early age.

A Mother's Journey to Natural Living

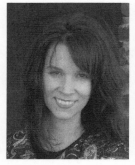

by Sara Elizabeth, http://www.AMamasStory.com

While I had a slight appreciation of natural remedies when I was younger, it was more of a feeling of awe and intimidation. I never imagined that one day I would successfully use natural remedies in my home and that they would work. In this chapter, I share my story of how the birth of my first child catapulted me into a life in which I questioned what I knew about health, wellness, and how to put my family on the right path.

"I want the shirt which reads, 'Drugs are good! Drugs are my friend!' I'm not afraid of childbirth, because I'm getting the epidural ASAP. And there's no way I'm going to breastfeed. Why mess with the hassle? The nurse told me there's absolutely no difference between breast milk and formula."

Yes, that was me almost eleven years ago.

My, have things changed.

Growing up in the Deep South of Alabama, I was no stranger to deep-fried food, whether it was fried chicken or fried zucchini. Then, due to inactivity after an injury my senior year of high school, I watched the number on the scale creep up. This lifestyle I led was giving me high blood pressure and high cholesterol while I was only in my mid-twenties. But not to worry, like several other Americans, I was brought up in a culture that believes there's a "pill for every ill."

Back then I never understood why folks didn't get to the doctor as soon as they had the tiniest sniffle. Didn't they know they were simply prolonging their misery?

When I learned I was pregnant with my first baby, I went to the hospital believing that everything would play out as it should. While I gave birth to a healthy baby girl, it was not the smooth sailing I imagined. Yes, the hospital staff responded to my requests, and I got the drugs I planned to receive but was not prepared for the amount of interventions that were to come.

Shortly after arriving to the hospital, my water was broken so they could insert a fetal scalp electrode for heart rate monitoring since her heart rate appeared to be dropping. Fortunately her heart rate showed stable with the new monitoring. Stating that my contractions were starting to space out, the doctor ordered Pitocin. As the intensity of the contractions grew, I was given more pain medicine through my IV and then Spinal Anesthesia. Soon, not only did I have external fetal monitoring and internal heart rate monitoring, but intrauterine monitoring was included to check to see if my contractions were really as strong as they were reading on the monitor. But while the baby's heart continued to remain stable inside the womb, she wasn't descending as quickly as I was dilating, and there was talk of a C-section.

Unable to move and hooked up to what felt like every machine possible, I felt helpless, terrified, and stressed beyond belief. All I wanted was to have my baby, but I felt things were spiraling out of control. Finishing off with an episiotomy, I did accomplish delivery without a C-section, but watching the resuscitation of my daughter immediately after birth is permanently burned into my mind.

I also was not prepared for such a difficult recovery. For the first day, I couldn't keep down food. For the first week, my baby had difficulty nursing, and I had zero confidence in my mothering skills or intuition. And just as we were getting ready to leave the hospital, as I literally could only shuffle my feet down the hall, I watched another new mother exit a nearby room, looking healthy, vibrant, and able to walk like a normal person! I learned that she had a very different birth experience.

And my life changed.

My first quest was to create a lifestyle plan. I wanted to ditch the diets and short-term exercise programs. I wanted something doable—something that I could enjoy for the rest of my life. So I talked with a holistically minded personal trainer who helped me make this a reality.

I also immediately changed the notion of "Diet and Exercise" as my focus became "Nutrition and Fitness." Finding an activity I enjoyed, I looked forward to doing it every day. I also cut out the sugar in my diet and slowly began to wean off processed and fast foods.

After introducing more whole grains into our meals and as my new habits continued, I noticed that not only was I losing my taste for white flour and sugar, but I was also losing pounds and inches, and dropping sizes left and right!

Once I saw real changes, I got radical and started reading up on herbs, alternative medicine, vegetarian and vegan diets, chiropractic care, and what seemed like the impossible: natural childbirth! I don't know why it didn't terrify me at the time, but I knew deep down that I could do it.

During the next pregnancy, I read as much as I could, hired a doula, stayed in shape, ate well, and after 36 hours of labor, naturally birthed my second child into the world. While 36 hours of drug-free labor may sound intimidating, they were easier than the 11 hours of labor with interventions I had with my first.

While I hadn't slept in 48 hours before his birth, I was able to function, able to eat almost immediately, and the baby nursed from the get-go. It felt so good to walk the halls of the hospital feeling well.

Had I arrived as a naturalist? Never! I'm always learning, so the learning has continued. Pushing me further on my journey, it turned out that my second child was going to throw me for a loop!

A few weeks after the birth of my second child, I developed postpartum depression. Since I was still new to the natural health world, I agreed to go on a low-dose antidepressant. While it was difficult to wean off of them, I don't regret taking them, as they were needed at the time. Eventually I met with a Naturopath, who introduced me to some natural alternatives, helped me wean off the drugs, and created a plan specific to my needs. (Note: Depression at any time is a serious issue. Please speak with a qualified care provider if you suspect depression or anxiety. I worked with both an M.D. and an N.D., while dealing with PPD.)

The supplements helped, and I continued to feel better. The Naturopath explained that the supplements I took were working with my body to help heal and treat an underlying cause, not simply treating symptoms.

But the big surprise regarding this child still hadn't come to fruition.

While pregnant with our third child, I watched a show about a family blessed with a special needs child. Not yet having had our ultrasound, I began to wonder about the baby in my womb and if the Lord would ever entrust us with one of these exceptional souls.

What I didn't realize was that He already had.

When my second child was about eight months old, his development came to a virtual halt. While he continued to grow physically, he simply wasn't with us; he was in his own world and wouldn't even acknowledge our presence in the room. We also noticed that he wasn't responding to his name, making eye contact, speaking, or behaving appropriately to sensory input—simply hearing the rain on the roof of our van would cause him to cover his ears and scream.

We soon had evaluations and started therapies. While these services showed progression, I knew deep down that we were missing something. We weren't treating the whole child. So we began seeing a chiropractor, researching diet, and talking to our Naturopath about herbs and other supports, such as digestive enzymes. We've not only seen great improvements in his development after implementing everything as a whole, but the maintenance continues as we've increased our knowledge to include the benefits of essential oils and homeopathy.

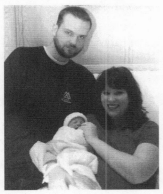

I guess you could say that while I mother my children, shaping and guiding them as I bring them up in the way of the Lord, they are also shaping and growing me, pointing me to ways that I believe He created to improve our health and life, and bringing our family back to the origins of His plan for us. They've taught me to trust the natural intuition I believe is given to me by my Creator, to see that the body is a miracle and how we can be destructive to ourselves when we consume processed food and/or unnecessary chemicals, and succumb to inactivity.

And so the journey continues! I never imagined I would eventually have a home birth, study Holistic Nutrition, or work toward becoming an Herbalist. While I used to see natural remedies as overwhelming and out-of-reach, in awe of those who were knowledgeable, friends and family now contact me for advice and suggestions when they need help.

Over the past eleven years, here's a list of the "Top Eleven" most important and practical things I've learned:

1. **Trust my intuition.** No one knows my babies better than I do. If something doesn't seem right, I shouldn't settle for a brush-off from an "expert." I can count many times when I've been correct

over a doctor. A couple of them have even recognized that, usually, mama is right.

2. **Always keep lavender, peppermint, tea tree, and eucalyptus oils on hand.** We use these items frequently. If you're interested in essential oils but don't know where to start, these are good ones for beginners.

3. As for Homeopathic tablets, **chamomilla is my go-to**, and I have reached for my Hyland's Kid's Kit on more than one occasion.

4. Before I felt confident enough to create my own tinctures and branch out with herbs, **I started out with the very basics**: chamomile, peppermint, nettle, oat straw, and red raspberry leaf. I use chamomile and peppermint for making teas when my family needs help with a queasy tummy. Nettle, oat straw, and red raspberry leaf are all nutritive herbs and my typical brew while pregnant.

5. **Use a daily probiotic**—find them in the refrigerator section of your local health food store. These are far more potent than ones you see on the shelf.

6. **Work fresh fruits and vegetables into your diet.** Children love smoothies and these are an easy way to get your daily servings.

7. **When possible, start weaning off white flour and white sugar.** I've learned that children develop both a taste for healthy and not-so-healthy foods, often depending simply on what they become used to eating.

8. **Don't underestimate the power of breastfeeding.** We practice ecological breastfeeding, so we breastfeed long-term and avoid pacifiers and bottles. I understand that not everyone wishes to follow this path, but the health benefits we've seen while breastfeeding extended beyond a year. I once heard that the benefits of breast milk do not continue beyond nine to twelve months. I simply don't agree with this statement. Research shows that breast milk certainly doesn't lose its nutritional value at a year. Contact your local La Leche League International for more information.

9. **Find an activity you can enjoy on a regular basis.** I believe this was key to getting control of my health. For example, running is a great way to drop weight, but if you hate to run, you probably won't do it consistently.

10. **Learn good nutrition and lifestyle choices to improve your health and that of your family.** Learn natural helps which aid your body in healing itself. Preventing illness is the key here, not waiting until you're sick.

11. **Check around your area to see if there are like-minded support networks.** These are helpful, especially if you have a good variety of both novices and experienced natural health practitioners to share ideas, remedies, and lifestyle modification strategies.

While the changes we've made over the years didn't happen overnight, our family is healthier now than ever. The changes weren't necessarily easy and we're not perfect, but it was worth the work. While we may use the occasional antibiotic or visit a conventional doctor when we feel it's needed, we are more knowledgeable and intentional about the decisions we make regarding our family's health care. I also want to add that if you feel that your child needs medical attention, please get it!

If you're interested in making positive changes in your life or your family's life, create some goals and find an Herbalist, Naturopath, lifestyle coach, etc. who can work with you. While books and other resources are fantastic for getting suggestions and ideas, nothing compares to having a person knowledgeable in their field, who can formulate a specific plan to reach your specific goals.

If you feel as though you've made too many bad decisions in your life to improve your health or your family's health, I hope that you'll feel inspired by learning how our family successfully made changes, step by step over the years. Changes didn't happen overnight within our family, but they did happen. Consistency is the key. Start small by changing dietary habits, choose an activity you enjoy, learn about a new herb, homeopathic treatment or essential oil each week and build your knowledge a bit at a time.

About Sara Elizabeth

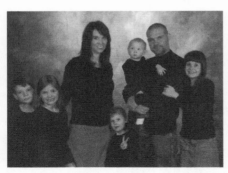 *Sara Elizabeth and her husband, Andrew, make their home in the Ozarks with their children. She enjoys writing about her family as they discover the joys of homeschooling, natural living, and strengthening their home through Biblical principles. A master herbalist-in-training, she enjoys working with herbs, essential oils, and using nutrition as a major part of preventive health.*

A supporter of Integrative Medicine, she understands there is wisdom in both natural and conventional medicine and has successfully treated minor illnesses at home, while knowing when it is time to seek out advice from a medical doctor. Learn more by visiting her blog, A Mama's Story (http://www. AMamasStory.com), to see how her family is "creating culture and breaking tradition."

The greatest joy in living lies, not in never falling, but in rising every time we fall.

~Nelson Mandela

Next up, hear from a CEO, Fashion Designer, and Mom who uses natural medicine to fight infection! Growing up her immune system had been damaged by a childhood filled with antibiotics. She had chronic strep throat, which brought her into the doctor's office, coming out with yet another prescription. Determined to keep her family away from her experience, she started to learn about natural healing. Her story is an excellent journey into finding what works for her and her family. She even shares her infection formula recipe!

Secret Go-To Infection Formula From
A Successful, Fashion-Designing Mom

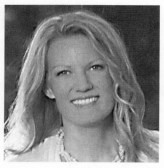

by Corinne Rickenbach, www.PersnicketyClothing.com

I have a long history of poor health, and I attribute that to antibiotics from my youth. Growing up I was constantly on antibiotics. My mother would put me on them for anything from a cough to my chronic strep throat. I was always at the doctor, and was always taking some form of antibiotic. I am convinced that this harmed my immune system!

When I was a teenager my mother began looking into natural remedies. Sometimes they would work, but my body had been so used to the antibiotics that most of the remedies wouldn't take. I was determined to get my immune system back on the natural track!

After I got married I started to really research natural medicine and homeopathic remedies. Then, when I got pregnant with my first child I knew I had to make some life altering changes with my diet. I just did not feel that we were eating as healthy as we should, or as we could! We started eating healthier, but by the time I had two children I knew I had to incorporate some new tools. My children would often get bad colds, coughs, stomach flu and ear infections. I started to look into essential oils, and I am so happy I did! I began seeing great results!

With my third child I developed Candida. I attribute this to my excessive antibiotic use from my childhood. It was so painful, and I was desperate to try anything that would help! I began a raw food cleanse, eating nothing but fruits and vegetables for a year. It cleaned my toxicity out and really helped with the yeast. However, it was probably not the best remedy while I was still breastfeeding. The toxins left my body, but my poor baby took some of them in. I would not recommend cleansing while breastfeeding!

Seeing the results from diet change and essential oils made me want to look further into these natural remedies. When I was living in Cedar City, UT I started to really look into using more herbs. I was a big fan of Dr. Christopher, and gained the knowledge I needed to start experimenting on my own remedies. I contacted Jenni Wilson (her husband was helping me with my chronic strep throat at the time) and she shared her Infection Formula with me. I was so grateful for this. Through my recently gained knowledge and techniques I learned from others, I was able to create my own formula. Now I feel naked without it!

Corinne's Infection Formula-Makes 2 gallons

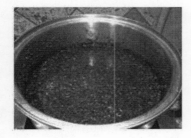

Measure 1/8 Cup of the following herbs:

- Echinacea root powder
- Myrrh powder
- Gota Kola powder
- Elderberries, powdered or coarsely ground
- Tumeric powder
- Astragalus root powder
- Yarrow flowers
- Cayenne powder
- 1/16 C Goldenseal powder

Combine the herbs with 6 cups of vegetable glycerin and let them soak for 2 weeks in a covered container (and up to 2 months).

Strain out half the liquid, which will remain uncooked.

Put the strained herbs and the other half of glycerin mixture into a pot with 6 cups of distilled water, and set the strained liquid aside. Simmer the herbs in the water for 20-30 minutes (cook longer for more potency), and strain. Put the strained liquid aside and put the herbs back into the pot. Combine 6 more cups of distilled water and simmer again for 20-30 minutes. Strain.

Use a new pair of panty hose to strain out the powders. Now combine.

I Love My Oils!

When any of my children show signs of getting sick I give this infection tincture to them. Usually, within 24 hours they are feeling better. This season my daughter got really sick. She was showing signs of pneumonia. She had spent the night at a friend's house the night before she started to get sick. They went swimming at night in the heated pool (during the winter), and then went swimming again in the morning. Soon after the swim they went ice-skating. Later that day when she was home she was just not herself. Within hours she became really tired and developed a high fever, along with a terrible cough . . . a really tight, painful cough that was not producing anything. I knew she was starting to get something nasty.

I turned to my Infection Formula and oils instantly, rubbing essential oil respiratory and immune blends on her. I also gave her ginger baths. After three days she was feeling better and began coughing up her infection! Had I not given her my formula and used these tools I am certain she would have been in the hospital.

During the sick season I rely on my formula as a preventative measure. We also like to do what I call "The Lineup": my children line up with their mouths open and I go down the line with a drop of my therapeutic/medicinal grade essential oil immune blend orally for each of them. As soon as they get their drop they run to get a drink! Most people do not like to take this straight, but we know it works, so we are willing to deal with the temporary unpleasantness. We have been doing this for so long that my children really don't mind the taste! One of my daughters actually begs for it all the time.

When health issues pop up, I am prepared! As I mentioned, we get our fair share of ear infections. My go-to method is melaleuca mixed with some olive oil. It clears up the infection in one day! When any of my kids feel the infection coming on, they *ask* me for the drops, because they know they will work. In fact, I have never given any antibiotics to my children for an ear infection. That is amazing!

Sometimes the stomach flu will make its way into our home, but we haven't had a really bad one in years (thanks to my formula!). To treat this I rely on my peppermint oil, and my essential oil blends for digestion and the immune system. I use them both externally (rubbing on the tummy) and internally (a couple drops in the mouth). They work wonderfully!

Last year not one day of school was missed! We are starting to really figure out which remedies work for us, and we've never been healthier. I highly recommend this natural lifestyle. It is the way our bodies were intended to be! Getting started can be overwhelming, so I'd like to share some tips for any newcomers.

First, turn your diet around. Try and stay away from dairy and gluten, and eat more fruits and vegetables. Get your body back to the natural state with a cleanse. This will kill off bad bacteria and rid your body of toxins. I would recommend starting with a colon hydrotherapy cleanse. This will prepare your body for future cleanses. Simply, when you do a cleanse your liver needs to dump out the toxins into your colon. When your colon is full of its own toxins, your body will back up. The toxins will have nowhere to go unless the colon is cleansed too. When your colon is clear, then your liver can adequately dump out the toxins, and they will be flushed from your body. You now will have a clean slate to start with!

Second, have some essential oils on hand, and learn what they can be used for. This is very easy to do, especially with the help of someone like Jenni. I keep my cupboard stocked with lavender, oregano, peppermint, lemon, orange, frankincense, melaleuca, and my blends for immune system, grounding and digestion. There are so many ways to use these by themselves or mixed together. They are very effective!

Third, use preventative tools like probiotics and an infection formula like mine. Once you find what techniques and recipe works for you, your formula will become your antibiotic! Another recipe I'd like to share is another preventative tool I use daily. I juice a lemon (and sometimes use lemon oil in there too) and put it in hot water with some agave or honey, cayenne and some stevia. It is a wonderful, and tasty drink to help cleanse your body and help fight off infections.

I am still learning and looking for new ways to live a healthier lifestyle. It is so important to have the right people to help you along the way. Learning about and incorporating natural remedies will become the best investment you ever made for your family. After all, nothing is more important that the health and well being of your loved ones!

About Corinne Rickenbach

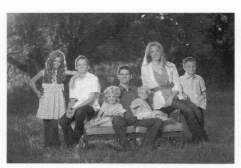

Corinne is an inspiration to so many people who are fed up with traditional medicine. Being a child of excessive exposure to antibiotics, her immune system suffered. She empowered herself by seeking help and guidance from natural remedies experts, educated herself on various techniques, and has been able to keep her family the healthiest they have ever been.

Corinne is a wife and mother of 5 active kids. She is active in her church and her children's many activities. She is the principle founder and designer of Persnickety Clothing Company, which offers "Fancy Little Frocks" for girls. As you can imagine, this keeps her very busy! You can occasionally hear from her on Persnickety's Facebook page and Blog.

If we could give every individual the right amount of nourishment and exercise, not too little and not too much, we would have found the safest way to health.

~Hippocrates

Coming up next is a girl who fought the label the conventional medical model gave her. Read the following story if you are interested in a woman's own health journey and how ultimately it lead her to the field of naturopathic medicine and ultimately to be a holistic mom. We all should be empowered to make changes so that we can achieve our greatest health potential.

My Change of Heart that took me from Medical School to a World Expert in Natural Medicine

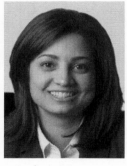

by Pina LoGiudice, ND LAC,
http://www.innersourcehealth.com

Many patients often ask me what "got me" interested in naturopathic medicine. Honestly, it is a story I love sharing because I want patients to know that my story is really no different than their own. We all have a health journey that encourages us to look inward, to look at the messages that our body, mind, spirit wants us to know, what changes do we need to make to move to the next level of our existence.

For me, the journey started at an early age. I recall I was about seven or eight years old when I began to notice how tired I felt and how often my belly used to hurt me. For years and years my mother took me to various conventional doctors with the hope of finding an answer, or at minimum, an explanation of why I was feeling the way I was feeling.

Unfortunately, most solutions were not helpful or had more problematic results. There was a point during this journey (I was probably closer to eighteen years old) when one physician plainly said during my visit "well, this is just what your body does and you have to just live like this." At that time, I did feel lucky I did not have a serious structural or fatal issue, but I felt this physician's comment to be insensitive, narrow-minded and that I was being dismissed. I think what bugged me even more so is the label he was trying to impose on me.

Regardless of feeling this way, I foraged on in the knowing that there still must be a better way. At some level, that doctor's words may have been the universe giving a guide to me—telling me to look elsewhere for health, and who I want to be. And with that I continued on with my college career at the University of Rochester. Being at University, I tried to live a normal life, but it was challenging.

While I enjoyed it so much, playing field hockey became more and more challenging as I experienced greater fatigue, and had digestive upset that left me unable to travel far from a restroom. Continuing on throughout college this way, it affected my social life and ability to enjoy the things most kids my age enjoyed. I could not risk being in a situation that did not have a bathroom within a minute's walk. Not the way a college girl wanted to live.

It only was after I graduated college and began my studies for the MCAT (the examination to enter conventional medical programs) did my life take an unexpected turn: while studying for this behemoth of a test, my mother knew how stressed out I was and suggested that I go for a massage to relax. Having never tried a massage, or any kind of 'alternative' therapy before, I thought I would give it a try.

I was fortunate enough to meet a woman that apparently practiced intuitive healing along with her wonderful massage skills. She asked me during the massage if I was experiencing particular health concerns of fatigue, body aches, and digestive issues. I was completely taken aback that a person had this ability to discern what was going on in my body without me explaining the situation. There is no way she could have known. Once I confirmed her suspicions, she recommended I see a "holistic nutritionist" further out east on Long Island from where I lived. I subsequently went home and told my mother of my experience.

My mother and I discussed having a visit with this holistic person (a term neither of us were familiar with) and decided to go for it. We figured I had seen everyone else under the sun, why not give it a try?

Not knowing at all what to expect during this visit, I was a little concerned of what it would entail. This holistic practitioner took an extensive history on all my health concerns (the most any person had ever asked me in years—certainly more than any doctor ever did). Then, he used his method of diagnosis I would learn later was called kinesiology. At the end of the one and half hour visit, he made several relatively simple dietary changes along with prescribing some herbal and vitamin formulations. I took the recommendations and supplements home, but was not sure what to think, or if it made any sense. My mother and I decided to take a leap of faith and have me follow along the recommendations given by this practitioner. None of the recommendations seemed dangerous, so what could it hurt?

Much to my and my mother's surprise and delight, within two weeks, I was a different human being. I hadn't felt incredible like that in years!! Energy abounded, and my digestive system was calm. I was absolutely astounded and amazed that making these minor changes and being educated on the food-health connection could create such profound change.

This was an 'aha' moment for me—I knew at that moment that THIS is the type of medicine that I wanted to learn and practice.

Following college, I took a position doing research as a fellow at the National Institutes of Health in Bethesda, Maryland. It was here I first learned about the profession of naturopathic medicine. When I discovered there were a few, distinct medical schools in the United States that taught the philosophy that "food can be your medicine and medicine your food" and espoused to its students that the body has the inherent ability to heal itself, I applied.

Being accepted to Bastyr University in Seattle changed the course of my life. While there getting my naturopathic doctor degree, I also received my masters in acupuncture. I truly cannot imagine working in any other than this profession. What a great joy and delight it has been for me to see the excitement in other patients when they too can remove the "sick" label that was stamped onto them. I know exactly what that feels like when a person walks in to my office for the first visit, and I know it is possible to change it.

During a naturopathic visit with my patients, I always discuss with patients the basic tenets of health. We focus on proper sleep, relaxation work and spirit (meditation/praying/de-stressing), drinking plenty of water, eating nutrient dense (preferably organic) foods and of course, exercise. The fact of the matter is that in our extremely toxic, energetically stressed out, nutrient depleted environment, it is more important than ever that my patients hold onto those tenets for dear life.

Most people may not realize this, but this is the first time in history that our children have a shorter life expectancy than their parents. A 2005 *New England Journal of Medicine* article revealed that children born that year would not live as long as their parents. Kids are getting adult onset diabetes in their early teens—something that also has never happened. If these are not the biggest travesties I have ever heard, I am not sure what are. And not to be pessimistic, I am truly not seeing the changes we drastically need to make in the world to reverse the profound decline in our health.

But, there is great hope too: British Medical Journal studies from 2011 confirm we can prevent cancer in almost half of people using lifestyle and diet changes. Other studies on genetics show that diet, lifestyle, not smoking, exercise, and living with less toxic load can prevent most disease.

So the greatest thing that I can do is impart on my patients the urgent need to hold onto those basic tenets of diet and lifestyle and natural health. While modern medicine is good at saving a life in time of crisis (like a car accident or heart attack), conventional care does drop the ball with chronic care and disease prevention.

We need natural health order to truly bring balance to our medical system.

The word doctor comes from the Latin word '*docere*', which means 'to teach.' It is my job to teach exactly how and why these natural recommendations work. Once my patients have a good grasp on the basics of health, then I will often encourage them towards specific botanical or nutrient formulations to help the body heal and repair too. Natural medicines are powerful and do work. They also enhance our own body mechanisms for healing and repair (unlike most pharmaceuticals, which will shut down mechanisms).

It is an honor to work with each patient in my practice and having seen the benefits of natural medicine in my own life, it is a joy to share it. It is my ultimate hope and goal that everyone can embrace the option of natural medicine and realize that our bodies do have the ability to heal.

I hope the story of my health journey inspires others to realize that they are more than any label ever given them. I would also encourage everyone to make appropriate lifestyle changes so that they may obtain optimal health and a great sense of well-being.

About Pina LoGiudice, ND LAC

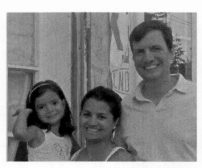

Hailed as a 'world expert' by Dr. Mehmet Oz on the Dr. Oz Show, Dr. Pina LoGiudice is truly a well-recognized expert in the field of natural medicine. Dr. LoGiudice graduated from Bastyr University, the leading accredited university for science-based natural medicine. Dr. LoGiudice is a co-author in the third edition of the Textbook of Natural Medicine and recently authored an original chapter on Pregnancy and Primary Prevention for the upcoming fourth edition of the Textbook of Natural Medicine.

*Considered a natural medicine expert, Dr. LoGiudice has been asked to appear on national TV (FOX), been interviewed on the Hallmark Channel, as well as been called upon as an expert on local television (**News12 Long Island**), radio (**Z-100's 'The Parenting Factor'**) and 'On the Air with Dr. Fratellone', 1600AM), and national web media (SustainLane, **Education. com**). Dr. Pina enjoys being a holistic mom, creating meals at home, and experiencing different cuisines with her husband Peter.*

The longer I live, the less confidence I have in drugs and the greater is my confidence in the regulation and administration of diet and regimen.

~ John Redman Coxe, 1800 A.D.

Alternative and natural treatments are not just for people, as you'll find out in our exciting next chapter. Turn the page to meet Laurie Driggers, an unconventional mom who helped to heal her four-legged boy Bruno by acting on her intuition, railing against a conventional diagnosis and pursuing alternative, unique treatment options that brought him back from a life-threatening medical emergency to living a life of health and wellness once again.

Saving Bruno: How I Used Natural Remedies to Heal My 4-Legged Baby

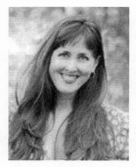

by Laurie J. Driggers, CHHC, AADP
http://www.inspiredhealthandhappiness.com

Nowadays, families come in all shapes and sizes. The children in our home run around on four legs instead of two, so our family is no exception when it comes to being unique. Caring for, loving, nurturing and protecting our four-legged 'kids' is a big part of my life and a responsibility that I take very seriously. Naturally, when one of them falls ill or is injured, I do everything in my power to make informed choices to help them to heal quickly and get back on the road to health and wellness. That is where my story begins . . .

It was a sunny day in May as I made my way to the 'beauty parlor' with Bruno, our lovable Pekingese, and his sweet little sister, Tweetie, our Japanese Chin, in tow. I normally groomed our babies myself, but our rugs were being shampooed, so I figured it would be a good idea to take these two little rascals on an outing for the day. With their chemical-free shampoo in hand, we arrived at the groomer's, and after a bunch of kisses and a couple good scratches, I was off for the day.

Several hours and errands later, I was back at the salon to pick up our babies. All seemed normal when I arrived until I saw Bruno. I immediately got a sick feeling in the pit of my stomach, as his eyes looked a little bit off. I noticed he wasn't wagging his tail in excitement to see me, which was normal behavior for Bruno and reunions. In that moment I brushed off my uncomfortable feeling and thought, he isn't used to the groomer's. He'll be just fine once we're on our way.

What happened next changed our lives forever. We walked out the door of the shop, and Bruno began to sniff around on a patch of grass. He lifted his leg to do his 'business' and fell over onto the ground with a heavy thud. As I bent down to pick him up, I noticed his eyes were glazed over and his tongue was hanging out of his mouth. I went into a complete panic mode while I picked him up and rushed him into the shop. Once we were back inside, I laid him gently on the floor and his convulsions started. The groomer said, "I think he's having a seizure." I felt the blood drain from my body. A seizure? I was in disbelief. He has never had a seizure before. He isn't even sick, I thought. "Call the animal emergency hospital for me and tell them we will be there in ten minutes," I exclaimed.

The trip to the emergency hospital was chock full of tears and prayers. Ten minutes seemed like ten hours on that short ride. When we finally arrived, the vet tech quickly took Bruno from my arms and whisked him away so that they could help him to stop seizing. Naturally, I had a million questions. Why did this happen? What does this mean? Will it happen again? The veterinarian did her best to allay my fears, telling me they would know more after some tests, and he would have to stay there overnight.

Overnight turned into three stressful long days before he could come home. When Bruno was stable and it was finally time for him to be picked up, I was told to prepare myself, as it would be quite a shock to see him and the physical state that he was in. Upon my arrival to bring Bruno home, I found he was quite lethargic and could not walk. I was told that they had found no definitive diagnosis for the seizures and that they could have been triggered by a variety of reasons, including a possible injury or even a smell.

"We had to give him Phenobarbital to stop the seizures," the emergency vet shared with me. Immediately I had another gnawing feeling in my gut. From what I've read about Phenobarbital, I didn't want him on that drug, as one of the possible side effects is liver damage. "He has never, ever had a seizure in his life, so I would rather he not be on this drug. When can I take him off of it?" I asked. "Bruno will never come off of it. He will be on Phenobarbital for the rest of his life. There is nothing that you can do about it," she said, looking me straight in the eyes.

That statement upset me. I was thinking that if Bruno were to be on it for the rest of his life, the rest his life wouldn't be very long. My motto is, 'there's always a way if I'm committed,' so I responded by saying, "With all due respect, I appreciate your opinion, but I don't accept your diagnosis. I *will* find another way. He will come off of this medication, period." There was an awkward silence, I collected Bruno, and we went home.

Seeing the state Bruno was in was absolutely gut-wrenching. His big beautiful brown eyes were dull and lifeless. He could barely move and would let out wails and screeches that cut into my heart like a knife. The vet said this was a side effect of the medication and would eventually subside, but it certainly didn't make it any easier to experience. As his mom I could not possibly let him stay like this. The Phenobarbital was only a Band-Aid, and we needed to get to the root of why he was experiencing the seizures in the first place so we could make sure they didn't occur again.

That caused me to begin thinking, what would I do in this situation if it were me? My answer was, I would look at my diet and lifestyle; what I had been eating, what had been going on in my environment, what therapies and practitioners could support me on my road to recovery. I, personally, choose to go to a holistic medical doctor, and now I wondered if they have holistic doctors for pets. I couldn't believe that I had never thought of this before. It truly makes sense that there would be veterinarians that treat with alternative therapies. I decided that I had some research to do, so I hopped on my computer in full detective mode. Within seconds, I found that there actually is an American Holistic Veterinary Medical Association. I felt as if a veil had been lifted off of my eyes and I could see a beacon of light beckoning me to follow it. I was elated, and now I had hope.

A few days later I made a phone call to my chiropractor to schedule an appointment for an adjustment. While on the phone, I explained to him what had happened with Bruno. He said, "Why don't you bring him to see me right away. I think I can help him." Well, you don't have to ask me twice. That awful feeling that I had felt in my stomach for the past few days turned into a feeling of knowing that I had surely stepped onto the right path. My chiropractor is a NUCCA specialist, one of only 400 chiropractors in the United States specializing in the upper cervical spine; specifically, the atlas bone. If this tiny bone that your head rests on is off even a millimeter, you can experience pain in your body. It can cause one leg to appear shorter than the other, and it can even cause you to walk crooked. I knew if anyone could help Bruno, he could.

It had been many days since Bruno experienced seizures and still he could not walk, so I carried him into the chiropractic office and gently placed him on the floor. After his atlas bone was checked, the chiropractor said, "Wow. I have treated many dogs in my career, and this is the worst I've ever seen. Bruno's atlas bone is wedged up against his skull. It appears he has sustained a trauma." I felt distraught that Bruno had been injured and relieved that I had some answers all at the same time. Another piece of the puzzle was falling into place.

What happened next was nothing short of a miracle. The chiropractor gently adjusted Bruno's atlas bone, and then Bruno stood up for the first time in days. I cried yet again; this time tears of joy. Huge waves of relief flooded my body as we left the office and I proudly walked our boy out to the car on his leash. Bruno was mobile once again, and we were making progress.

Before I left his office, I mentioned that I had a great idea to find a holistic vet to help Bruno restore his health and get off the Phenobarbital, but I hadn't had any luck in securing an appointment. My chiropractor told me he knew of a well-regarded holistic vet in our area that happened to be accepting new patients. I took down the information, and with one quick phone call, Bruno was able to be seen the next day.

Walking into the holistic animal hospital for the first time was like receiving a beautiful warm hug. It felt as if we were meant to be there. When our new holistic vet, Doctor Chris, shook my hand and promptly picked Bruno up to give him a snuggle, I knew that my intuition was correct. We were definitely in the right place and in the right hands.

After introductions were made, I nervously told the tale of what Bruno had been going through over the previous week. I talked and talked, and Dr. Chris patiently listened, which I find is the sign of an amazing holistic practitioner. Since clear communication is the key, I let him know that my ultimate outcome was to get Bruno off of the Phenobarbital. My first question was, "Is it possible to get Bruno off of this medication?" "Yes, it is. Don't worry, Laurie. Bruno will be just fine," was his reply. I knew by the look on his face and the certainty in his voice that he meant it.

Doctor Chris explained to me that one of the ways he treats his patients is by utilizing Traditional Chinese Medicine, so the first thing that he did was check Bruno's tongue. Upon inspection, he shared with me that his tongue appeared greasy and was a color that meant that our boy was 'out of balance.' "We need to get him back into balance," he said, which made sense to me.

Because Bruno appeared anxious being in a new environment, Doctor Chris used lavender essential oil to calm him down. A dab on his nose and on the inside non-furry parts of his ears did the trick. He relaxed, which also made me relax. I was delighted that he used essential oils, because I utilize them in my daily health regimen also. I didn't realize that I could use these with our babies, too. Great information, I thought.

Now in a calmer state, Bruno was ready for his first acupuncture treatment, which works by balancing the energy meridians in the body. The treatment lasted about a half hour, with adjustments being made by adding a needle here, subtracting a needle there. I was amazed that he didn't seem to be bothered by the needles and actually appeared quite relaxed. By the end of the session, Bruno was visibly more comfortable than he had been in over a week. Next came a chiropractic adjustment, which also went very well. This adjustment focused on Bruno's spine, not his atlas bone, which was 'stuck' in a few spots. After the adjustment, we both noticed that he definitely moved around the room better.

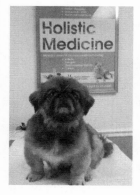
By the end of his first appointment, Bruno had a treatment plan, and I had some changes to make at home to play my part in Bruno's healing. Bruno would be treated with acupuncture, chiropractic and orally with medicinal Chinese tea pills that would support his liver and prevent further seizures from occurring. He was to be given homeopathic medication and herbs for pain. And the biggest change was that I would be preparing homemade whole-food meals for Bruno based on Traditional Chinese Medicine to help bring his body back into balance.

I found this all to be very exciting and also very daunting at first. It was going to be a lot more work for me because I was used to setting a bowl of dry organic dog food out for him to eat. Now I would be in the kitchen preparing his meals.

Over the months that followed, Bruno was seen weekly by Doctor Chris as we continued with his treatment plan. Every few weeks, after rechecking Bruno's tongue and reassessing his health, I would come home with new tea pills and a new list of foods to prepare that would further restore his body to balance. It all worked like a charm. Bruno's journey began in May and ended in October when he received his last dose of Phenobarbital, something that I was told was 'impossible' by conventional medical standards.

By forming a partnership with our holistic veterinarian, we had gotten to the root of the issue, which was an imbalance in Bruno's body, instead of covering it up with a Band-Aid, the medication, which would surely have led nowhere that we wanted to go. It truly was spectacular to watch Bruno's transformation from a dog that I thought was literally going to die, to becoming his happy, tail-wagging self again. If I hadn't listened to, trusted and followed my intuition, our boy may not be with us today.

Although it was a painful experience to go through, today I am grateful for all of the events that occurred, as all of the lessons that I learned and the knowledge that I gained was priceless in being able to keep the little members of our family healthy and happy now and into the future.

About Laurie Driggers

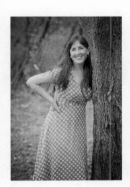

Laurie J. Driggers is a board certified Holistic Health Coach, a Living Light Culinary Arts Institute Living Foods Chef, and a Healthy Living Expert. Through her online eHealth coaching company, Inspired Health & Happiness, she works with women worldwide, empowering them to discover how they can live a balanced lifestyle by truly nourishing both their minds and their unique bodies. She passionately uses her experience and knowledge to inspire and motivate women while they create healthy and happy lives that they love by sharing with them her own health secrets, tips for holistic living and whole foods cooking expertise.

*Symptoms, then are in reality nothing
but the cry from suffering organs.*

~Jean Martin Charcot

Learn next from Robin Konie how to let the real you shine through, with natural solutions to acne! This woman discovered that the real road to healing her skin was by taking her health into her own hands. While frustrated with dry and acne-prone skin, this woman was looking for answers in all the conventional places. Unsatisfied with her doctor's response, she dove into a world of natural health that proved to be life changing.

Taking Health Into My Own Hands: How Acne Brought Me Gratitude

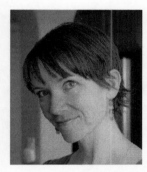

by Robin Konie, http://www.ThankYourBody.com

Most days I think I live a pretty normal life. My house is nice and clean (I mean toxic free). My food is nice and clean (just toxic free). My body is nice and clean (just toxic free). Sensing a pattern here?

My dad calls me a hippie. I don't get that. I mean, I don't have long unwashed hair that's parted down the side with twigs or flowers in it. I don't bob my head around like I'm in some sort of crazy daze.

The truth is I just feel more grounded, relaxed, healthy, and energized by the very things other people think are "weird." And if you are comparing my day-to-day living to that of a "normal" person . . . well, I am weird. Or at least different.

Of course, I didn't start this way. I grew up in a "normal" home with good parents, lots of processed foods, over the counter drugs, and the usual issues that come with both.

Even though I didn't grow up in some sort of hippie community farm, I have always been interested in health. In my youth I would set goals to eat less candy, exercise more, and reach an "ideal" weight. And yet, despite my attempts at being healthy, I struggled with acne, digestive issues, and weight problems. Even during my college days when I was dancing 8+ hours a day, in addition to working out, I continued to feel trapped in someone else's "not quite right" body. I wasn't sick, but I sure didn't feel at my peak.

During those college years I had also experienced severe dry skin on my hands. Seriously, I felt like a leper. I would pour piles of lotion and frown as it just pooled in my palms. It was useless. This condition continued to come and go for four years. FOUR. **YEARS.**

I finally went to a doctor to see what was wrong. His diagnosis: Dry Skin. His recommendation? Put some lotion on it.

Frustrated, I went home and started researching. I spent hours online, reading chat forums, nutrition journals, and other people's experiences. After a lot of consideration I determined I had an omega-3 deficiency. (Keep in mind this was several years before omega-3's would be a "buzz" word. Nobody I knew had ever heard of omega-3 anything.)

I bought some flaxseed oil supplements and began my self-prescribed plan. Within a week or two my hands were back to normal. I soon traded the supplements for omega-3 foods (What do you know? Fat can be good!). It has been 8 years and I haven't had a problem since.

This was a pivotal moment for me. I learned four important truths:

1. Many doctors far too often only address symptoms, not real issues.
2. The body uses a lot of different means to get our attention. My dry skin was my body's way of saying "I need help!"
3. Most importantly, we **must** take control of our own health.
4. More often than not, there are more natural approaches to healing than our society believes.

I want to talk mostly about number 3 and 4.

Our Health Is Our Responsibility

Any journey toward real health must start with the realization that our health is our own. Instead of waiting for answers from those who too often only cover up symptoms, we need to take the steps necessary to get back to basics. We need to see that health care is not the same as sick care. Health care is an ongoing and **vibrant** process, a personal journey.

What does that mean to me? Does it mean never trusting my doctor or always going against modern medicine? No, not necessarily. But it does mean not necessarily putting my whole trust in them without trying to learn, research, and considering all my options. It means using common sense, seeing a bigger picture of health, trusting my gut, listening to all sides, and doing what feels best.

After curing myself of my "dry skin," I started looking for natural remedies to better my health as much as possible. That's not to say that I think all pharmaceuticals are evil, I just believe that often the thing to cure us can be found in more simple things. Moving, nutrition, de-cluttering, de-toxing, etc—these things help lead us to real health (All without negative side effects, too).

Annoying Issues Remind Us of Natural Healing Power

As I have continued on my journey I can say with a full heart that I am grateful for my body and grateful for those shifts in perspective that have brought me to this place. I am thankful that I wasn't willing to accept my doctor's "diagnosis" and that I dug a little deeper and found a more basic approach to healing. You know what else I'm grateful for? My acne.

This is actually a difficult thing for me to write about. I have struggled with acne since I was 11 years old (I'm in my thirties now). It was a constant source of frustration and embarrassment. I never went anywhere without makeup on. Dance became my sanctuary because the only time I felt beautiful was when I was onstage and the focus was off my complexion.

I had tried all sorts of "stuff": over-the counter creams, prescription drugs, online remedies, etc. In high school my mom had the dermatologist put me on birth control, which just made me crazy (and I will never use again, thank you very much)! Thankfully, I avoided Accutane, but only because my older brother had such a horrible experience with it.

I remember once during my freshman year of college looking online for some sort of solution to my skin woes. I was getting desperate and it seemed my doctor couldn't fix my acne. Maybe some sort of "miracle" treatment online would do the trick.

Once again I found myself sifting through natural approaches to healing. During my research, I came across an article with the statement **"why you should be thankful for your acne."** By this point I was nearing my mid 20's and was sick and tired of feeling like a greasy teenager. In a bitter tone I said sarcastically, *"Oh yeah, I am sooo thankful for my acne."* Still desperate for solutions, I continued to read the article. The main point being this (*very* much paraphrased):

Be thankful for your acne. It's your body's way of telling you something isn't right. Most of us are experiencing ill health due to poor nutrition and unhealthy lifestyles. Some people are "unlucky" enough to not show symptoms, riding some "genetic inheritance" that keeps their skin perfectly clear. Be thankful that your body is sending you a message to change."

This article didn't make me stop in my tracks, but I had started my journey . . . even if I wasn't aware of it yet. Eventually, step by step, I moved closer and closer to the way our bodies were designed to connect to the world. Changes came in my movement and diet. I started giving up our toxic cleaning supplies for homemade "green" versions. My husband finally convinced me that I was beautiful without my makeup so I gave that up, too (mostly). I tried to listen to my body, moving it and energizing it.

I just started to "let go" of all those things our society, doctors, and drug commercials tell us we **need**. I trusted the wisdom of those who lived before our lives were cluttered with products, fads, and chemicals.

This gave me the courage to trust my body. It gave me the courage to trust nature. It gave me the courage to look for answers beyond symptoms.

Dry skin and acne don't really seem all that monumental, but seeing how modern medicine approached it, helped me see that there are better ways. Now, as a mother, I utilize the power of real food, herbs, essential oils, and other time-tested natural remedies first. In fact, I have yet to really "need" modern medicine for my family yet. That's not to say that I'd turn it down if the circumstances merited their use. I believe good can come from our modern medications. Although, with their array of side effects, they should be used sparingly, indeed.

It's important to do your research. Talk to experts. And trust your gut. Our health is not something to be placed at the bottom of our priority list. If we take care of our bodies by trusting the natural laws that govern them, we can find a transformational experience that will help us shed away the layers of issues, problems, and challenges that our modern world sees as "a part of life."

Getting Back to Basics, Back to "Me."

Not too long ago, I was talking to my husband about this whole transformation that I wasn't really trying to make, but that happened anyway. The words that came out of my mouth surprised me, but got to the core of what I was feeling: "I finally feel like the *real* me is out. The me that I always felt was inside, but that nobody else could see."

This is the power of basic health. When we strip away all the clutter, trends, and guilt and then give ourselves time to refocus, go back to basics, and respect the wisdom of the body/nature, that is when the "real me" is able to come out. For someone who always struggled to feel beautiful, for the first time in my life I *knew* that I was beautiful. I also realize that there are probably lots of people out there who feel the same way I did: trapped under layers of "not me." When we live in a world that tells us synthetic chemicals and products are necessary to be beautiful, we know something is wrong.

So in the end, getting back to a natural approach to health isn't really about being a "hippie," it's about being what I was ultimately designed to be.

Have you often wondered what the "real you" looks and feels like? Don't be afraid to strip away all the garbage that the world, modern medicine, or anyone else says you need. Within our bodies is a natural capacity for healing, for health, and for true radiant beauty. Take matters into your own hands and discover the wisdom of your body.

About Robin Konie

Robin Konie writes at ThankYourBody.com. She is a Registered Somatic Movement Therapist (RSMT) and a Certified Laban/Bartenieff Movement Analyst (CLMA). With a deep passion and respect for the human body, she has been exploring ways to help others reclaim their personal power and embodied way of knowing through movement, nutrition, and holistic approaches to health. With an MFA in Modern Dance, Robin has taught dance and somatic-based classes at Brigham Young University. She has also taught for the internationally recognized Integrated Movement Studies Programs. Robin continues to learn and grow as she works with clients through individualized movement therapy.

It is no use saying we are doing our best.
You have got to succeed in doing what is necessary.

~Winston Churchill

In the next chapter, Rachel discusses how the body functions and heals, and how God created our bodies to heal themselves. Have you ever heard that idea before? She doesn't take lightly that during emergencies she is thankful for conventional medical treatment, but for non-emergencies she shares 3 easy steps to living a more natural lifestyle. By incorporating these steps, they can help you on your own journey. Her quest to use her intuition and common sense, has helped to keep her family healthy.

Maximize your Living!

by Rachel Marie, http://www.day2dayjoys.com

Mom's carry all kinds of labels.

We're homemakers, housewives, mothers, stay at home moms, working moms, and we all have one goal in mind. We want the best for our families. We want our families to flourish, to be happy and healthy.

For each of us mothers there have been many a time or two that we used our intuition to guide us. We've had a weird feeling about letting our child go over to so-and-so's home. For me when I had a newborn, I was feeling pressure from doctors and others to medicate or vaccinate my child when something in me told me that wasn't right for **our family**. Your intuition gives you a gut feeling that you know is right even when everyone else is telling you you're wrong.

Our switch to a more natural lifestyle came while my husband was pursuing his Doctorate, while I was finishing my bachelors and we were broke students. My husband was learning how the body works, that God created you from one cell from your mother and one from your father. By 6 weeks, your brain and spine were created which then create the rest of your body.

While he was learning all of that I got pregnant with our first child, I started thinking about what I was putting in my body more and more and how we would raise this baby. I had grown up in a classic American family, we followed the typical medical model, when we got sick we took some medicine, we ate the SAD (standard American diet) diet, we never used any natural remedy and to me this was the norm, why would I choose anything different for our child.

191

After our son was born I felt pressure a couple of times from well-meaning loved ones to give him Tylenol for a low grade fever. My intuition was telling me, along with my husband, that this was the wrong choice, but being a young mother I was easily influenced. I wanted the best for my baby. They were telling me it was okay, so I did it.

Let me back up to what my husband was learning in school. He learned that after 2 cells got together and created you, 9 months later you were born. God put this amazing power to heal into all of our bodies. So if you cut your finger while dicing some carrots for dinner, a couple days later a scab will form, and a few days after that, your finger will be healed. You didn't need anything; your body healed it for you. God doesn't make junk.

When my son got a fever, he wasn't deficient in Tylenol. His body was fighting an infection in his body. Fevers are a good thing. Let me repeat that. **Fevers are a good thing,** and now I know my intuition was right. I did not understand this at the time and society definitely does not teach this. What we hear is that if your child has a fever they need to go to the doctor, or you need to give them medicine. And that just wasn't the route we felt was right.

Our society and most of the medical community just wants to label problems then cover them up with a medication, a surgery or a procedure. If you break a bone, if your child gets a fever or any other sickness or disease, our bodies were made to heal themselves.

All of our bodies have a nervous system that controls every function, tissue and organ in our bodies, for you to breathe, for you to birth a child, for you to even be reading this right now, the information travels from your brain down your spinal cord out through all your nerves and has to get to the right place. My husband, a wellness chiropractor gets so passionate when he is teaching this concept, because it is so simple. If you are having a health-related issue, it could likely be because you have interference in your nervous system.

"The power that made the body, heals the body."—BJ Palmer

After learning this truth about health and healing we made it our mission to help educate our community and empower people to know **that they are in charge of their health**. To keep my family happy and healthy, the first thing I do is make sure everyone is getting regular chiropractic adjustments. Thankfully we have Dr. Daddy. Then we focus on eating real foods, getting exercise, and removing toxins, along with having a healthy mind.

Since the Tylenol incidents, our son and our daughter have never been to the doctor, they have never been vaccinated, nor have they ever had a prescription. We have had our share of sickness, intense fevers, teething discomfort, ear infections, and rashes, but my first inclination has never been to get them checked by a medical doctor. When one of my children is sick, the first thing we do is a chiropractic adjustment to create an immune response. Then I'll look for a natural remedy, such as honey for a sore throat or cough, or tea tree oil for a rash.

Now, here is what I know for sure. Some folks just don't believe in chiropractic care. **The good thing for us is that chiropractic is a proven 117 year-old science**. And the truth is simple. The brain controls the body. Remove interference between the body and the brain, and the brain will heal the body.

My husband recently shared with me a study of maintenance care patients, and it stated that Chiropractic patients spent only 31% of the national average for health care. It also concluded that maintenance chiropractic patients had 60.2% fewer hospital admissions and 62% less outpatient surgeries. That's proof that it works. When I make chiropractic care a priority, I am stewarding over my family's health by raising the next generation with tools designed to keep them healthy.

In 2012, there was another study conducted in Germany that concluded 80% of all children have **"Blocked nerve impulses at the top bone in the neck (C1)"** which can **lower resistance to infection,** especially ear nose and throat infections. This means that their bodies are stressed and burdened by misalignments. If your children have never been checked by a family chiropractor, it's time (JMPT 2012).

Now adjusting the spine won't help if your finger is cut off, so if there is an emergency, we are thankful that we live in America with the best emergency care in the world. Last year I had an ectopic pregnancy, and if left untreated, it could have been life-threatening. And even though I wasn't happy to get shots and blood tests, I was thankful that I had the care I needed.

Recently our son was injured from a falling piece of playground equipment. The biggest question you need to ask yourself is, "Is this an emergency?"—when you are feeling overwhelmed with a sick child, illness or accident. As for us, we sat it out for the day, watched our son, made sure he wasn't lethargic, and that his pain wasn't unbearable. The next day, as much as we try to avoid seeking medical intervention, my husband did take him to friend who is an MD. The second opinion was reassuring. Although he did not prescribe anything, it was nice to hear that our son was okay on the inside.

You may be thinking, well that is easy for her to say all of this. Her husband is a doctor. While that is true, there is a group of doctors that are teaching these same principles, who have caring hearts, are very family oriented and make care affordable, no matter your income. I would suggest a wellness family chiropractor or better yet, a "Maximized Living" doctor.

*"The doctor of the future will give **no medicine**, but will interest his patients in the care of the **human frame**, in **proper diet**, and in the **cause and prevention of disease**."—Thomas Edison*

My husband is a Maximized Living doctor and we teach 5 essentials of health and healing. I have been very fortunate to walk alongside my husband and see lives and families transformed by these essentials, and by living a more healthy, abundant life.

Essential #1: **Maximized Mind:** Understanding the true principles of health and healing, and creating a mindset of success

Essential #2: **Maximized Nerve Supply:** Restoring and maintaining proper function of the nervous system through spinal correction

Essential #3: **Maximized Nutrition:** Nutritional science that sustains well-being, disease prevention and ideal weight

Essential #4: **Maximized Lean Muscle and Oxygen:** Cutting edge exercise that allows your body to take in higher levels of oxygen and creates lean muscle that keeps both your body and mind healthy

Essential #5: **Minimize Toxins:** Supporting the body's own ability to permanently remove toxins from cells

You can find more about these essentials here: www.maximizedliving.com

Once you have made a decision to live a healthy, more natural lifestyle, stick with your guns. Educate yourself, do your research, use your intuition and don't ever let anyone bully you into making a decision you do not feel is right. First try natural remedies before using conventional medicine and take baby steps towards healthy lifestyle changes.

Some of my favorite tips to living healthier life are so simple and frugal that they are easy baby steps to make. And remember, if you are trying to switch to a more natural lifestyle, please take it one day at a time.

Here are three baby steps to consider making:

Eat Real Foods

I'm sure you've heard of the saying "You are what you eat." If you are eating processed foods, artificial foods, loads of refined sugar, aka man foods, undoubtedly you are experiencing a wealth of health issues. So not only is eating this food causing harm on the inside of your body it can be costly to your wallet and is grounds for medical problems like obesity, inflammation, diabetes, cancer and more.

Our bodies were created to eat God food, not man food. God foods are whole foods like: fruits, vegetables, herbs, nuts, seeds, beans, lentils, whole grains, and healthy fats.

Try Natural Remedies

If you are experiencing an illness, rash of some sort, fever or other sickness that is not an emergency use your intuition. Do some research and try a natural approach. I know this can be scary when making a switch to natural lifestyle.

Let's talk about immune systems for a minute. Immune systems are like Olympic athletes. An Olympic athlete doesn't train for only 2 or 3 weeks out of the year. They are battle tested and trained. They train for years just to get a chance. But because of their hard work, they got better, faster and stronger. Why would the immune system be any different?

Our immune systems need to be battle tested through exposure to different things, such as bacteria or viruses. When one of our children gets a fever, tummy ache or headache (which is rare), the process is simple, natural and safer than traditional medicine. Providing adjustments, removing sugars, serving clean foods, insuring rest and including prayer. Then if it continues for a couple of days we may give them Vitamin D3 or a silvercillin supplement. Because we do this, we notice that our children are rarely sick more than 24 hours. I do want to say that we aren't perfect; we have just found a system that works.

Here are some of my favorite natural remedies I use in our home:

- **Fevers**—luke warm bath, lots of rest, love and liquids
- **Dry skin or eczema**—coconut oil
- **Headaches**—peppermint essential oil on temples
- **Sore throat or Coughs**—raw honey
- **Rashes**—tea tree oil
- **Bug bites**—paste made with baking soda and water
- **Chiropractic adjustments**

Reduce Toxins

There are so many toxins around us including environmental, household, food and life factors that it is impossible to remove all of them. You can get caught up in this and that and the other which can be very overwhelming. My suggestion is that you start by making small changes, then once you are comfortable with them, start making some more.

Toxins to learn about and reduce:

- **Food**—It is vital to survival, right? So it's the first thing you want to investigate and learn about. Start by learning how to read food labels and eliminate MSG (monosodium glutamate) a neurotoxin. Then remove anything artificial, especially artificial sweeteners since they have been connected to horrific side-effects, and recent studies suggest they cause cancer. *Switch to real foods and if you can't read it (the label) don't eat it!*
- **Plastics**—These contain phthalates and our bodies are unable to naturally detoxify them which causes damaged hormone receptors, altered brain chemistry, can lead to learning disorders, ADHD, and can cause cancer. *Switch to stainless steel and glass.*
- **Cleaners**—Your skin soaks up everything to which it is exposed to whether it's skincare products or cleaners, all the toxins contained in these products go inside your body. *Switch to homemade cleaners and use coconut oil for lotion.*

This is just a little part of my story and the different steps we've taken to live a naturally focused life. God intended our bodies to be able to heal and if you take the right steps to eat a balanced diet, to maintain a healthy nervous system, exercise and reduce toxins in your life, you will start to feel healthier and will be able to live a more fulfilling life.

About Rachel Marie

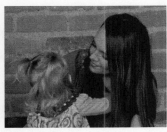

Rachel is a mother to 2 children and a wife to a wellness doctor. Her passions are faith, family and health. She supports her husband in helping to change the way people look at their health and uses her blog, www.day2dayjoys. com, as a tool to do that. Her husband also has a feature on her blog called, "Ask Dr. Jake".

He would be happy to answer any of your health related questions or at least direct your path to some better options.

You can find Rachel writing about her family adventures, encouragement and inspiring you to make healthier choices for your family and more at day2dayjoys or on Facebook.

Epilogue

By Jenni Wilson

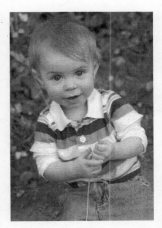

When my 7th child was almost 2, I had the **scare of my life**, and it gave me a greater appreciation of each moment I have with my children. I had just arrived home from dropping 2 kids at birthday parties. It was 7 PM, my son had prepared some dinner, but nobody had eaten yet. I scooped up my smiling toddler, Ian, walked straight to the pot of food (our healthy version of mac and cheese) and gave him a big bite. He chewed for a moment, and then started choking.

He had eaten a big bite or possibly two in a row, so I just thought he hadn't chewed it enough. I moved to the sink, draped him over my arm and tried to do the Heimlich maneuver. He didn't cough anything out and wasn't breathing well. His eyes started fluttering and that's when I knew something was really wrong.

I yelled to my 15 year-old Boy Scout son to come quick and continue doing the Heimlich while I called 911. They told me they were sending paramedics and continued to ask me for details. My older son had been unsuccessful in helping Ian, so I took him back and by this time, he was limp in my arms. He was semi-conscious, but he wasn't turning blue. I held him very still and could hear that he was barely breathing.

My husband is an ER doctor and probably could have resolved the problem in seconds, but he was working 45 minutes away at the time. My son had been unable to reach any neighbors by phone. He was so scared and frustrated that he ran out to the street and started yelling for help. I was still trying to do the Heimlich and talk to my baby to keep him fighting. He was struggling greatly to breathe.

Luckily, it didn't take that long for the paramedics to arrive. I told them I thought he had food in his throat and needed suction. They quickly tried to suction him, but nothing was coming out. I was trying desperately to keep Ian coherent. They put a monitor on him and could tell he was getting a little oxygen. They tried to give him some through a mask, but it wasn't helping.

The paramedic then put some instrument down Ian's throat. The next thing I knew, he had pulled a little bouncy ball out and was holding it in front of my face. Relief washed over me. Even though my baby Ian was still semi-conscious, I knew he would be okay.

At that point, Ian had been struggling hard to breathe for about 15 minutes. Something came to my mind that I had learned from a recent class about how essential oils can help get oxygen into the body. I immediately ran to my storage case of oils on my kitchen counter. I grabbed peppermint, frankincense and a grounding blend. I rubbed a few drops of each on the bottoms of his feet and chest. One of the paramedics commented after a few minutes, that the oils seemed to be helping increase Ian's oxygen levels.

My paramedic neighbor arrived ready to help, and was happy to see that the main problem had been resolved. We decided to take Ian to the hospital in the ambulance so he could get stabilized with extra oxygen and get checked out to make sure he was fine. Before we loaded him, I asked my neighbor, who is a member of my church, to give him a blessing. He did so, and between the essential oils and that blessing, I was completely comforted and calmed.

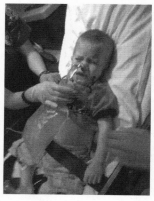

On the way to the hospital, Ian started responding again. They pricked him for something and he cried, which was a response that made me happy.

I looked at my older son, and he acted as if he might lose his emotional control. I had a key chain on my purse, which held essential oils, so I handed him a bottle of a calming essential oil blend. He just sat in the ambulance, smelled the oil for a few minutes and then was fine and even smiling.

At the hospital they did a chest x-ray, and could tell that Ian's lungs had taken a beating. They said his oxygen levels were pretty stable though. I had some of a respiratory blend of essential oils in my key chain as well. I carry small, sample size bottles that usually have a dropper piece, but that one didn't. So when I went to apply a drop to Ian's foot, I dumped out the whole thing onto the hospital bed. It was fine because then he could just breathe in the healing, strengthening aroma.

I realized that it was 8:30 or 9 PM by then, and Ian hadn't eaten anything for a while. I asked for something and got apple juice and graham crackers. After Ian ate and drank, he perked up much more and started laughing and playing. He seemed to be getting back to normal.

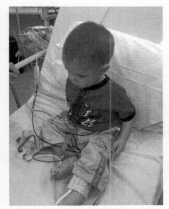

A respiratory therapist came in to give Ian a treatment. The treatment uses steroids to reduce inflammation. I generally try to avoid them, but in an emergency, I would definitely use them. I just wasn't sure they were really necessary by that point. The nurse had commented that Ian's oxygen was good, so I asked the respiratory therapist if he thought it was good. He said yes. I told him I didn't want the treatment then. He said okay and walked out.

The ER doctor, who was a personal friend, said he was a little worried about Ian, and normally might keep him overnight to make sure he did okay. I was so happy that he just kept us there an extra hour, and then let us return home. It definitely would have cost us to spend the night.

Because we have a high deductible insurance, I had to pay the hospital before we left. It was $2000, $300 for the ER visit, $100 for the radiologist fee for looking at the x-ray and $1600 for the ambulance ride (which was billed to us later). I was doubly glad then that I had used my essential oils and had declined the respiratory treatment. Conventional medical treatment is expensive!

When we arrived home, I pulled some of Dr. Christopher's Respiratory Massage oil out of my natural medicine cupboard and used it to dilute more essential oils for Ian before putting him to bed. We checked on him that night and he was fine. He showed no signs the next day that anything had happened.

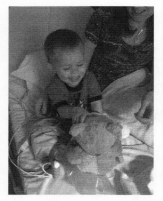

As I reflect on this experience, my feelings and gratitude about a few things are solidified. I am so thankful for caring and well-trained rescue teams, nurses and doctors who save and improve lives. I'm also thankful for the technology that helps them with crisis management. This is where conventional medicine shines and I consider it to be a great blessing that we have it.

I recently met a surgeon, Dr. Joshua Yorgason, who is looking for natural healing solutions, such as essential oils, to help patients avoid taking drugs with side effects and perhaps avoid needing surgery. He feels that natural medicine can help patients become more grounded and in tune with their inner sense of health and wellbeing, and to decrease their dependence on drugs.

Dr. Yorgason and other professionals launched http://www. protocolled.com. On this website, professionals can subscribe to natural treatment protocols which have been written based on the medical literature and on their own experience with patients. Dr. Yorgason says that patients who follow these step-by-step regimens and complete the surveys will not only help validate the treatment, but through this process of self-awareness and self-testing, they will become comfortable with the natural products and will know how to use them to help improve their medical condition.

I am immensely grateful for natural tools that can increase our wellness, many times preventing crisis, and often healing and strengthening after a crisis. Synthetic drugs can help greatly during a crisis. They can manage problems, but because they are made from isolated, unnatural compounds, they often carry negative side effects. They almost never heal, balance, strengthen or nourish the body.

Natural tools like herbs, essential oils and even whole foods do nourish, strengthen, balance and heal the body in many different ways. Whole foods should be at the foundation of our health if we want our health to be good. Natural solutions can be used for fine-tuning, wellness and comfort. But these tools are powerful enough to heal and manage many illnesses, when used correctly. Their regular use can often prevent situations from ever getting to crisis point.

My fondest hope is that we can all learn about and obtain natural healing tools for our homes, such as whole, foods, herbs and essential oils.

It is empowering. It helps us be more self-reliant and confident in a world with many voices about "how things should be done."

Dear readers, thank you so much for your interest and for reading all our experiences! We hope they empower you! We wish you the best of luck and blessings in your health, and happiness in your lives and families!

Get Jenni's Free Video eCourse on Hardcore Principles of Health!

- ◆ Learn more about the differences between natural and conventional medicine
- ◆ Understand how drugs differ from nature's solutions
- ◆ Hear how processing of whole foods makes them unnatural and unhealthy
- ◆ Discover more about natural tools for wellness
- ◆ Get educated on the different ways to use natural medicine

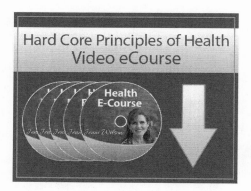

Go to http://www.NaturalMedicineMom.com to get your free videos now!

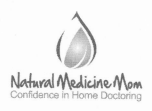

Are you seeking for alternatives to toxic, synthetic drugs?

Subscribe to the

Becoming
Doctor Mom

Home Medicine Academy

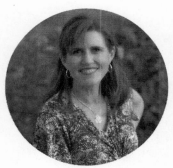

--------------- **STOP** ---------------
Wasting hundreds of dollars on doctor visits
& feeling helpless during illness!

--------------- **START** ---------------
Empowering yourself with the NATURAL
and SAFE tools to regain control
over YOUR family's health!

ACCESS JENNI'S CLASSES!

**Strengthen your confidence in healing from home!
An AWESOME VALUE for life-changing information!**

Your investment for
Becoming Doctor Mom: Home Medicine Academy is
ONLY $1 for the first month, then $10 per month after that!

Unconditional 30-Day Guarantee!
Register at http://www.BecomingDoctorMom.com
To your home medicine empowerment!

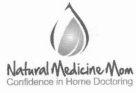

Natural Medicine Mom
Confidence in Home Doctoring

4655196R00121

Made in the USA
San Bernardino, CA
01 October 2013